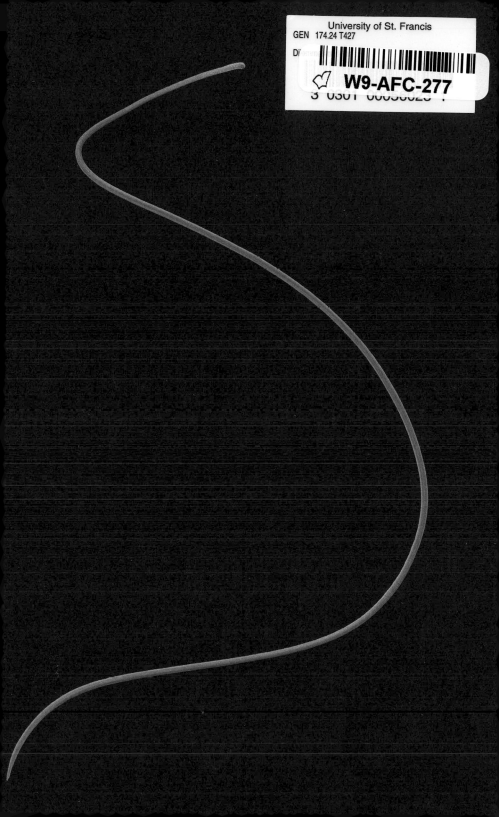

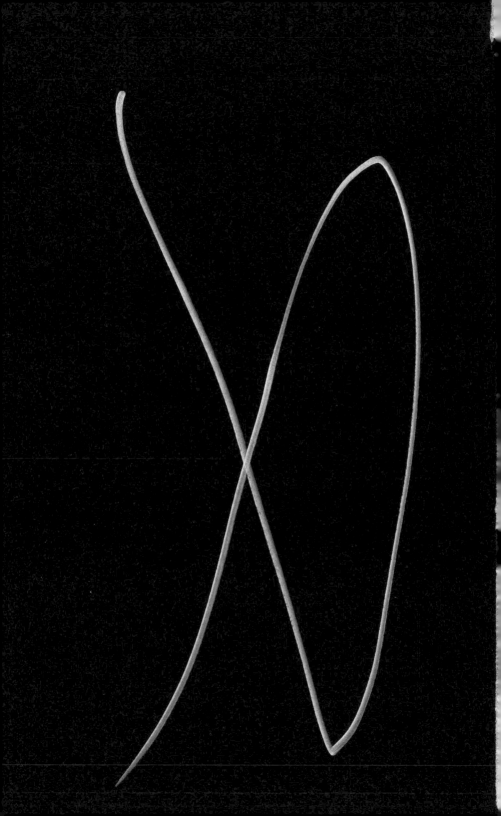

Edinburgh Medical Group

MORAL ISSUES IN HEALTH CARE

1

DILEMMAS OF DYING

a study in the ethics of terminal care
edited by
IAN THOMPSON

EDINBURGH
at the University Press

© 1979
EDINBURGH UNIVERSITY PRESS
22 George Square, Edinburgh

ISBN 0 85224 367 7 (hardback)
0 85224 378 2 (paperback)

Printed in Great Britain by
T. & A. Constable Ltd., Edinburgh

174.24
T427

CONTENTS

99288

Preface

MUCH OF THE value of this report lies in the original and distinctive nature of the experience which it seeks to encompass. Such an experience can hardly be summarised even at the length of this report, it is almost impossible for it to be shared. The group whose work is the subject of this book was convened with three thoughts in mind. First, that members of the medical and caring professions often mishandle the all-too-human ethical and emotional problems involved in tending the dying and the bereaved. The idea was that these common misjudgments have their roots in 'professional' attitudes and practices, sanctioned over the years with the authority of habit. The first task of the group, therefore, was to expose instances of such misjudgments, and of the ethical dilemmas which they entail. The method was to assemble representatives of the medical and caring professions, and give them ample chance to be frank about their own feelings and attitudes—either in direct exchanges, or in commentary on case studies. The hope was that *the members of the group*, simply by 'being themselves', would provide the necessary evidence of the roots and nature of the difficulties under consideration. This hope was, I think, largely realised, as readers will discover.

Its realisation leads to the second thought: that difficulties in 'managing' the dying and bereaved would be greatly lessened if the relevant professionals could effectively communicate their differing perceptions, values and attitudes, and coordinate their aims and approaches. Put like that, it sounds simple! But, again, the care with which the group was selected and assembled ensured a wide range of attitudes and experience—and hence heightened the problem of effective communication. I would say that, whatever their opinions two years ago, no member of the group would now under-estimate the challenge of communication and coordination. The measure of mutual understanding and respect eventually attained took time and effort. Perhaps it cannot be otherwise.

Which leads again, to the third thought: these problems could be greatly eased by more suitable professional training. An appeal to 'Education', of course, is often the last resort of the desperate: but the hope remains that exposing trainee doctors, nurses, social workers, ministers, and so on, to the dilemmas of caring for the dying before their 'professional' habits and attitudes form a protective emotional shell around them will lead, given time, to a more sensitive approach to these matters. So the group had not only to explore the problem area—but how it might be remodelled and remapped, and future explorers retrained.

This approach and method has many implications, of which I will mention just two here. First, it shaped my role as Chairman, and hence (inasmuch as that role had any effect) moulded the experience of the group. In discussion of medical matters, I am a 'sympathetic outsider': my main concern is with the training of natural scientists, and my frame of reference (broadly) sociological. From time to time, I could enter the discussions as a participant. But I took my main role to be to attempt to help the members of the group to be open, frank and honest with each other. Being a 'chairman', my intrusions were usually camouflaged as attempts to achieve 'clarification': but sometimes the clarification was pursued in order to peel away what I suspected was a complacent consensus, and so expose underlying *conflict*; while at others its object was to *reduce* conflict by eliciting a position around which consensus might re-form. Groups being what they are, I spent more time trying to expose conflict than remove it! Anyone who contemplates training future professionals in matters so complex and value-laden as those tackled by this study group must be prepared to *work* to bring conflicting values and assumptions to the surface: for the polite conventions of society discreetly paper over such cracks—and it is the helpless, the dependent, the dying and the bereaved who can inadvertently suffer in consequence. If trainees cannot be helped to appreciate such conflicts (within themselves, as well as with others) *before* they find them exemplified in 'real life', their chances of avoiding the misjudgments of their elders must be lessened. We can no longer afford to opt for 'easy ways out'.

Second, this study group's report cannot be expected to follow any conventional pattern. To attempt a detached, 'objective' style would be to throw away the central, involved, revealing and *educative* core of our two years' experience. To us, the experience was *itself* an education; we wish others to follow a similar path, and share similarly educational experience; we therefore feel it necessary to *reproduce*, on paper, as much of that experience as possible—so that readers can appreciate its 'flavour' and 'texture'. Since what we 'discovered' in our 'research' was so closely tied up with the particular individuality of the group, the report can only do justice to the experience by reproducing that particularity—much as a novel seeks to impart *general* insights by a minute inspection of individuals.

One thing is clear: the problems to which this report draws attention cannot be resolved merely by finding time, in medical training, for a new 'subject' to be added to the syllabus—and called, presumably, 'Ethical Dilemmas in Dying and Bereavement'. For one thing, the appropriate method for exploring ethical dilemmas bears little or no relation to that appropriate to the exposition of the contents of Gray's *Anatomy*. But, more importantly, if these ethical dilemmas are to be realistically face d whole patterns of institutional behaviour demand scrutiny, and probably modification: habits and values must be painfully exposed and questioned. And this is a challenge to the whole structure of the medical and caring professions. It cannot be confined to those who write and agree medical curricula, and to the students who sit respectfully at their feet. So we commend this report to all who share our concerns—professionals, students and laymen—to read and ponder. The reader can decide what specific course of action it calls for, given particular circumstances. The report lays down no hard-and-fast rules. Do not do as we *say*—do as we *did*. Or something roughly similar . . .

David Edge

Research in Medical Ethics

MEDICAL ETHICS stands in need of new definition. It is still associated with the kind of medical etiquette which evolved during the last century as Physicians, Surgeons and Apothecaries sought to clarify their relationships with one another and with the patient public. The stereotype of medical ethics as concerned with the size of doctors' brass plates and their relationships with female patients still holds for many. The publicity given to the activities of the General Medical Council when a doctor is struck off the register reinforces this view as primarily concerned with excluding quacks and censuring conduct prejudicial to the good name of the profession. 'Medical Ethics' undoubtedly encompasses such issues within its meaning, but it is not limited in its scope to a code of conduct for members of the profession.

The Hippocratic Oath and other more modern equivalents, which seek to define the moral responsibilities and professional duties of doctors in general terms, point to another aspect, which is concerned with maintaining proper standards of confidentiality, respect for the life and dignity of patients. This aspect is concerned with the nature of the relationship between the doctor and patient and the definition of the kind of moral framework within which that relationship should be conducted. The Hippocratic Oath is typical in emphasising both the aspect of loyalty to the medical fraternity as a self-regulating professional body (professional code) and the duties and responsibilities of the doctor to maintain the highest standards of patient care (the doctor-patient contract).

The formulation of more recent codes and declarations by medical bodies has been provoked by both technical developments and improved therapeutic possibilities of medicine on the one hand and the abuse of medical science in the interests of warfare and political ends on the other. The Nuremberg trials and the revelation of the atrocities of Nazi medicine and experiments in eugenics, provoked the formulation of the *Declaration of Geneva* 1947, as a modern restatement of the principle that a doctor has an obligation always to act in the best interests of his patient, to act to preserve human life, to maintain secrecy on matters of confidence and to give emergency care in the absence of others capable of doing so. Other declarations have been provoked by the need to clarify the scope and limits of medical responsibility in the light of new scientific developments e.g. human experimentation (*Declaration of Helsinki* 1964), therapeutic abortion (*Declaration of Oslo* 1970), ethics of transplantation (BMA *'Consent to Treatment'*) and determination of the moment of death (*Declaration of Sydney* 1968).

The technical and scientific developments which have caused a re-examination of the moral issues involved in the practice of medicine, have also produced a situation where a considerable number of para-medical technicians, research scientists and specialists with particular skills such as occupational therapists, physiotherapists, social workers, psychologists and ministers have become involved in health-care. In addition, nursing has become both more specialised and diversified as a profession, and nurses exercise an increasing degree of responsibility in patient management. The result is both a blurring of the boundaries of clinical responsibility and a need to clarify the scope and limits of responsibility for each of the professions involved in health-care. Some of the most urgent problems of medical ethics resolve into problems of communication and problems of demarcation of the boundaries of responsibility, and in that sense come back to the questions of etiquette and the definition of codes of conduct in the various professions—which preoccupied the Victorians.

In Britain, the development of the National Health Service with associated raised expectations of an improvement in the standards of health-care, has meant increased public and government interest in the problems. The media treatment of moral dilemmas in medicine and the availability of information about modern developments in medicine have created a body of public opinion increasingly concerned about the moral issues raised by the practice of medicine. The proliferation of groups and organisations concerned with the study 'medical ethics', 'bio-ethics', and 'values in health-care', (e.g. the various Medical Groups in the U.K. linked through the Society for the Study of Medical Ethics, the U.S. Institute of Society, Ethics and the Life Sciences, The Kennedy Institute of Bioethics, and the Society for Health and Human Values) and a growing literature in the field suggest that medical ethics has acquired a new importance and broader meaning in the context of modern health-care.

If medical ethics is seen as the study of moral issues raised by the practice of health-care, then it is obvious that it is not the kind of subject which is either the exclusive preserve of doctors, or of any other individual profession. The issues are of concern to doctors and nurses, to social workers and ministers, to administrators and government departments, and the general public.

An 'Aristotelian' approach

Medical ethics challenges us to find an appropriate point-of-view from which to approach the questions it raises about the exercise of moral responsibility in health-care and the proper attitudes, values and goals which should direct practice, planning and policy.

The social sciences may be relevant to clarify and assess what attitudes and values are. The techniques of psychological and sociological survey would yield useful descriptive and statistical data about current views. These sciences could also provide invaluable historical information on the origin of professional codes and the social determinants which have moulded and made them what they are. The social and behavioural sciences could also give us vital information about the socio-economic and psychological context in which moral decisions have to be made in contemporary health-care. However, these sciences could not, without being unfaithful to their ideals of scientific neutrality, help us to decide or evaluate ethical questions.

Medical ethics is concerned with the practical exercise of moral responsibility in real-life clinical circumstances, with decision-making and riskful value-judgments. It is unavoidably concerned with normative and prescriptive questions and not merely with the description of how things are; with 'ought' questions and not merely 'is' questions. As a normative and cultural science it would seem to be most appropriately studied by the analytical and logical methods of moral philosophy. However, moral philosophers by and large do not have the necessary knowledge and experience to appreciate the niceties of moral judgment in clinical situations. Because what is demanded is primarily practical moral wisdom, rather than theoretical knowledge of different belief-systems and how to justify logically one's ultimate moral beliefs, the philosopher alone is not able to provide what is required to help resolve some of the practical moral dilemmas facing professions involved in contemporary health-care. The knowledge and experience of the doctor needs to be supplemented by that of nurses and other health-care professions, and all need to be complemented by psychological insight and knowledge of the sociological forces at work, as well as the analytical insight and clarifications of value-judgments and the notion of obligation which moral philosophy

xiii

provides. All this argues the need for a multi-disciplinary approach to the study of medical ethics.

In search of an appropriate method we might turn to the origins of our Western tradition of moral-philosophy, in the moral dialogues of Plato and the ethics of practical wisdom advocated by Aristotle. These men lived in a period of unprecedented moral and social change not unlike the situation in modern society and in medical ethics in particular, as Greek society faced up to the changes from a rural to an urban and commercial civilization and confronted the relativities of different social customs and moral values in the expanding Hellenistic empire.

The methods involved are those originally suggested by Socrates for the clarification of moral issues, namely, the critical interrogation of the experts and sustained public and rational debate, aimed at reaching a public consensus in the clear identification of the issues and the definition of the criteria appropriate for deciding them. This approach agrees with the spirit of Hippocrates who insisted that 'every physician should be a philosopher', that is to say, that he should constantly be engaged in the critical reappraisal of the attitudes and values on which professional practice is based. (Thompson, I. E., 1976)

Aristotle spelt out in detail what such an approach entailed. First, ethics should start from an examination of existing moral attitudes and proceed from these to the clarification of fundamental principles and criteria. (Aristotle: *Nichomachean Ethics*, I)

Ethics should be based on the study of the actual moral
judgments of men of experience . . . . men of general
culture . . . . versed in the practical business of life.

Second, the orientation should be practical: 'Ethics is a study the end of which is not knowing so much as doing.'

Third, the method should be appropriate to the subject-matter and should not pretend to a greater degree of precision than is possible. Ethics is not mathematics.

In studying this subject we must be content if we achieve as
high a degree of certainty as the matter of it admits . . . .
we must be satisfied with a rough outline of the truth, with
broad conclusions.

Fourth, the goal we aim at is a sufficient degree of public agreement for co-operative action to be possible and the interests of justice to be served. Moral judgments are 'objective' to the extent that they rest on a public rational consensus, and are open to revision and criticism on the basis of further knowledge and experience.

On this model, research in medical ethics would start with an examination of the ordinary moral judgments of doctors, nurses and other health-care professionals in the context in which they operate. It would require an approach which is case-based and directed towards the clarification of actual decision-making.

The Form and Purpose of the Report

The Report falls into three parts: Part I, The basis of professional involvement with the dying and the bereaved; Part II, Case-based studies of areas of moral conflict and dilemma; Appendixes, Practical implications and recommendations.

Part I represents a summary of how the multi-professional Working Group attempted to define how and why health-care professionals should and do become involved in terminal care and care of the bereaved. In the course of examining present practice a number of key areas of moral conflict and dilemma were identified—the basis and justification for professional intervention in terminal care, the scope and limits of patients' rights in terminal care, the question of the right to die, the conflicts experienced by the professional between conscience and professional duty, conflicts of values in inter- and intra-professional relationships, the dilemmas relating to the limits of professional responsibility illustrated by anxieties about the medicalisation of bereavement.

These six areas of moral conflict and dilemma are illustrated in the case-based discussions in Part II. Each chapter has a similar form: Introductory statement of the problem, summary of the main points discussed in the chapter, case-presentation, illustrative discussion, and analysis of conclusions. Each chapter is intended to stand on its own as an example of our method of doing research in medical ethics, as an example of case-based multidisciplinary discussion of a central moral dilemma in the care of the dying and the bereaved, and as a tentative exploration of some of the theoretical issues which emerge from these studies. For example, the discussion of the ethics of intervention in terminal care led to critical examination of the limitations of the concept of contract in medical ethics; the discussion of patients' rights to the examination of rights in general and the right to die in relation to euthanasia and suicide; the chapter on conscience and professional duty to the discussion of moral dilemmas and practical strategies for dealing with them; the chapter on conflicts of values in inter- and intra-professional relationships led to discussion of responsibility and accountability in institutional contexts; and, finally, the discussion of the risk of medicalisation of bereavement led to the discussion of the limits of professional responsibility and the professional's wider social responsibilities.

xv

Introduction

The appendixes attempt to spell out the practical implications of this study and to offer recommendations for the improvement of professional training for care of the dying and the bereaved, and to offer some practical suggestions for the improvement of day-to-day practice.

Preliminary Reflections on Professional Attitudes to Death

This study project was launched by a weekend residential conference on 'Death and Professional Ethos' in which some thirty medical, nursing, social work and divinity students participated. The reasons for beginning with students were twofold. The project had been initially conceived and sponsored by student members of the Edinburgh Medical Group. It was felt that students could bring a critical, non-institutional point-of-view to bear on the subject. The vividness of the questions asked and the problems raised by the students confirmed the value of this approach.

The attitudes of health-care professionals to death and bereavement are not entirely independent of the attitudes prevalent in society at large. The fact that death is not around like it used to be was cited as a likely cause of our being able to cope less well with it, and the feelings and anxieties it provokes. The changing pattern of mortality—with a dramatic decrease in infant mortality rates, the reduced proportion of deaths among younger people, and the general increase in life expectancy—has led to a situation where most people can reach middle age without having experienced the death of a close relative. The fact that most dying is done by the elderly and the elderly tend to live in relative isolation and obscurity on the periphery of society, means that death itself tends to be more hidden. This obscurity of death has contributed in part, it was suggested, to the 'conspiracy of silence' about death in the community.

The popular stereotypes represented by death-on-the-media reinforce images of death which are epidemiologically untypical. Sudden, accidental and violent deaths, which account for a very small proportion of all deaths, assume a disproportionate significance in the public mind and serve to over-dramatise the role of medical staff in life-saving acute medicine. The media also perpetuate the image of cancer-death as the symbol of a death which is necessarily painful, prolonged, distressing and degrading—in spite of the advances in terminal care and particularly the use of drugs. Again, the fact that cancer accounts for less than a quarter of all deaths and that respiratory and cardiovascular diseases are the greatest killers has hardly penetrated public consciousness (Cartwright et al, 1973). The ordinariness and undramatic character of most deaths is not appreciated by the public and medical and nurse training is not geared to dealing with typical death either. These factors seem to have something to do with the social attitudes which make relatives put pressure on GPs to hospitalise dying patients and account for the slow progress in the development of domiciliary care and community-based services for the dying.

It was suggested that popular expectations of science and technology and a more materialistic approach to life make it more difficult for people to accept the inevitability of death. This in turn results in strong social pressures on the doctor to preserve an optimistic approach : 'the last thing we will allow him to do is to die'. There is a consequent unwillingness on the part of most medical staff (except perhaps in geriatric medicine) to admit that death may be desirable or that it is necessary 'to settle for comfort'.

The medical students insisted that these attitudes tend to be reinforced by medical training. In general it is assumed in Medicine that life is always better than death. *Death is the enemy*. Medicine is seen as a struggle against death, and medical training is seen as training for this battle. The death of the patient tends to be seen as a defeat. There is reluctance to admit that there may be some fates worse than death—chronicity, dementia, loss of dignity. The concentration in training on acute, hospital-based, high-technology medicine reinforces the image of the doctor as the knight in shining lab coat doing battle with death surrounded by ministering 'Angels'. The low prestige associated with the treatment of the chronically ill, mentally and physically handicapped, and geriatric patients was, it was suggested, associated with 'the attitude of medical failure in the face of living death'.

Students said that their own personal attitudes to death might have a significant relation to their choice of medicine as a career. They considered that this might have something to do with the defences doctors build around this area and the fact that doctors, as much research has shown, tend to back away from too direct involvement with the dying. (cf. Feifel, Herman et al, 1967 and Peretz, David et al, 1971).

Doctors first learn about death differently from other health-care professionals—namely in the dissecting room. The strength of personal reactions from students suggested that many were profoundly affected by this experience. They remarked on the strangeness of the fact that the first patients they encountered were cadavers which they were expected to dissect, and the fact that they had to develop defence mechanisms to enable themselves

B   xvii

to cope—the attempt to reduce dissection to a purely technical business, the contrived informality, macabre jokes, chatting to friends and eating sandwiches over the dead body. The formal emphasis on the details of physiology and anatomy to the exclusion of anything personal was seen as part of the serial desensitisation of medical students to the facts of death. The ability to distance himself from death and dying by escape into the purely technical mechanics of medicine might be helpful to the doctor, but whether it was helpful to the dying patient, or in dealing with relatives, was seriously questioned.

In contrast the exposure of nurses to death is very different. Nurses emphasised that they have plenty of physical contact with live patients e.g. in feeding, washing, dressing, shaving, etc. They are allowed to touch people in a way that is not generally acceptable except in the context of intimate relationships, particularly the relationship of mother and child. For this reason it is easy for the nurse to develop an intimate and confidential relationship with the patient, but more difficult to escape from the reality of the dying patient or to remain emotionally detached. The emphasis on efficiency, on keeping nurses busy, might be necessary means of defence for the staff, enabling them to cope with the experience of death on the ward ; but this could have the unfortunate effect of isolating the patient, preventing the nurse from maintaining empathic contact. This was particularly likely in a task-orientated rather than patient-orientated regimen of nursing. The advantages to the dying of continuity of care from those who have developed an intimate relationship with them were readily admitted but it was pointed out that nursing routines frustrate this possibility and nurse training neglects its importance.

The experience of 'laying out' the body of a deceased patient was mentioned as a significant experience for the nurse-in-training. While one student nurse maintained that it had a traumatic effect on her and adversely affected her subsequent attitudes to the nursing of dying patients, the more general opinion was that it was most helpful in assisting the nurse to face the reality of her own shock and bereavement and the ending of a relationship with the patient—especially where the patient had been on the ward a long time. The significance of 'giving the last rites' was seen to consist in 'doing and giving something for someone you have cared for and respected'. 'It is a means of completing one's task in relation to the patient almost in a ritual sense.' (Medical students remarked that they lacked this kind of opportunity to conclude their relationship with patients.) The act seemed to emphasise continuity, that life processes move on. The performance of these last rites by the nurse in the home could have special significance to the bereaved family.

In general practice the experience of death was seen to be very different from hospital death and while district nurses have necessarily had to be trained to deal with death in the home, the doctor comes to general practice unprepared for it. He is not taught in the course of his training to cope with death in the home and its consequences. Unlike the hospital doctor the G P has usually known the dying patient for some time. This has advantages and disadvantages for doctor and patient. On the one hand the G P is often as reluctant as the family to admit that the patient is dying, and appropriate terminal care is often delayed. On the other hand, while the hospital doctor tends to feel out of it, death is not the end-point, but the centre-point of a process in which the G P is involved. It is perhaps easier for the G P to cope because he has a role both before death and after, in caring for the bereaved. However, facing bereavement may be more difficult than facing death and the G P may find it easier to get alongside the dying patient than his relatives—especially when anticipatory grief makes the relatives very critical of the doctor.

Doctors are ill prepared to deal with the highly emotional area of peoples' reactions to their own impending death or that of a close relative. In particular they find it difficult to discuss prospective death where general degenerative processes and mental deterioration are involved, and easier when death is a clear probability in relation to a definable illness. The concept of death as a relief can be very acceptable after death has occurred, but people find it difficult to accept beforehand because of the guilt which may be engendered by the realization that the relief may be greater for the caring relatives than the patient. There is for both doctor and relatives the fear of criticism that not all is being done that might be done. Proper co-operation in terminal care requires careful preparation of all involved.

The students agreed that Social Workers' training, particularly the study of different reactions to loss, provided them with a greater willingness to look at relationships with a less exclusive concentration on the patient's body and medical complaints. This enabled them to cope better than other professionals with the complex emotional problems which arise in dealing with chronically ill patients and terminal states, if and when they become involved in these areas. Doctors, it was said, are set on winning the battle against disease and death, however, you don't 'win' relationships. Social workers and nurses, it was argued, are better able to cope with death and dying because they are not set on winning. Curing is the prestige aspect of medicine, whereas social work in general is concerned with helping people to cope. *There is not much curing in the dying process.* Doctors and even nurses have difficulty admitting the limitations of technical medicine, when the problem is to help people to cope with the inevitable. Social workers are better equipped by their training and experience to assist people who are dying or suffering from some chronic physical disability or mental illness. Few social workers, however, are attracted to work in these areas because most social workers want to work with children.

The potentially vital role of the social worker in coordinating and channelling the resources of the community to help a family nursing a dying relative, and in co-ordinating support to the bereaved, particularly isolated and vulnerable widows, was recognised, but it was felt that in training and practice these functions of the social worker are given low priority. Social workers bear some responsibility for the fact that death in the community remains a hidden area of distress.

Theological students were particularly critical of the fact that while ministerial training ought to prepare clergy for a more realistic approach to death, in reality it does not. Ministers frequently have no experience of death and bereavement before they are confronted with the responsibility of conducting funerals and consoling bereaved relatives. The lack of practical experience of death procedure, ignorance of the problems and tasks faced by undertakers, even lack of training in how to conduct a funeral or how to cope with intense grief, mean that newly trained ministers are ill-qualified for ministry to the dying and the bereaved. The tendency of such ministers to take refuge in pious platitudes and a theology of denial was remarked upon. Nevertheless, the emphasis in pastoral training is changing e.g. with hospital placements, and that a more realistic theology of death and training in ministry to the bereaved is changing things for the better in some centres. The fact that many dying patients request to see a minister and that virtually all funerals are still conducted by clergy at the request of relatives was seen as significant, not so much as evidence of concern with matters of religious faith as confidence that ministers are familiar with death and know what should be done. Religious rites and ceremony, it was felt, satisfy the feeling that things should be done decently and in good order.

PART ONE

Professional Involvement with the Dying and the Bereaved

ONE

Pre-Death and the Professionals

THE CONSPIRACY of silence which surrounds the dying and bereaved is not only the result of public attitudes which have made death a taboo subject, but also due to uncertainty and confusion in the minds of health-care professionals regarding their role in terminal care and care of the bereaved.

Attitudes to death, on the part of the public or professionals, embody different values, which are founded upon different beliefs about the significance of human life. As researchers have shown, attitudes to death have varied considerably from one epoch to another, with changes in religious beliefs, in social conditions and, more recently, in the effectiveness of medicine. The modern attitude, which Aries (1976) calls 'forbidden death', is the result of family and society attempting to protect the dying patient from the ordeal of dying and to protect themselves from the effects of having to contemplate the death of a loved one. The consequent tendency to hand over responsibility to the hospital, which Ivan Illich in *Medical Nemesis* (1975) has described as the 'medicalisation' of the problem, is the inevitable result of the tendency to treat death as something private and forbidden. (Cf. Gorer, G. 1965; Choron, J. 1973; Boyd, K.M. 1977). There is a consensus that public attitudes today prevent a frank examination of death and bereavement, lead to a conspiracy of silence around the dying and to the isolation and stigmatisation of the bereaved, encourage the abrogation of responsibility for terminal care to professionals, and discourage the frank and critical examination of the scope and limits of professional roles and responsibilities in this field.

What is evident is that the issue of professional responsibility for the dying and the bereaved cannot be discussed adequately without a corresponding examination of such value-laden questions as: what constitutes a good death, what are the duties of professionals and what are the responsibilities of the family and society? The conspiracy of silence can be broken and the ethics of terminal care clarified only if these questions are seriously discussed and examined.

In Part I of this study an attempt is made to explore these

2

questions as they arise in concrete situations, in the hope that this will illuminate the kinds of value-judgments which have to be made in particular cases. This case-based approach represents an attempt to avoid the temptation of imposing global interpretations on these questions which will pre-empt the debate about the ethics of terminal care and the meaning of death and bereavement for contemporary society.

We begin by identifying a number of areas of moral conflict and dilemma for professionals involved in terminal care. In the following three chapters we discuss these issues in relation to the three different phases; Pre-death, Death and Bereavement. In this chapter we consider two problems central to the involvement of professionals in the pre-death phase: the basis of self-justification for the doctor involved in terminal care; and the problem of defining Pre-death, as a basis for professional intervention in terminal care.

The right to intervene, by a Physician

The patient approaches the doctor and asks for medical attention, often under the duress of fear and acute personal need. The involvement of the doctor at this stage tends to extend naturally into the management of the terminal stages of an illness, without re-examination of the pre-suppositions on which the implicit contract between doctor and patient is based. In normal circumstances the doctor undertakes responsibility for the treatment of the patient in the initial stages of an illness and then continues his management through the phase when recovery or alleviation is expected, into the phase when death is imminent.

There are two kinds of situations in terminal care where doubts and uncertainties can arise for the doctor in the exercise of his medical role. These relate to the doctor's activity or lack of activity a) when the patient is at the point of death, i.e. when death is likely to occur in less than 48 hours; b) when the patient is old, suffering from severe and distressing disease, including dementia, which means that he is unable himself to instruct medical attendance. Here the concept of distress is an important criterion for medical intervention as it introduces the patient's variable reaction to the stress of his circumstances, including the human and physical environment round about the patient. The fact that the patient may have to be nursed in poor circumstances, for example, may alter the management of the case.

The legitimacy of the doctor's position may be questioned in three kinds of circumstances: a) when the patient is unable to express a wish for intervention; b) where the doctor feels it is incumbent on him to pressurise the patient i.e. when the patient does not know the range of possibilities and explanations may be long, complicated and specialised; c) when the doctor departs from what the public regard as his remit, namely, to preserve life at all costs. In such circumstances, when the doctor is obliged to act on his own initiative, his self-justification for intervention is based on general beliefs about the value of life and health-care

Such beliefs about himself allow the doctor to act in the conviction that he is right, and morally justified in what he does. He bases his judgment on more than strictly medical knowledge and expertise. His confidence in his own goodness and the good of medicine is reinforced by the trust of patients, the public and other staff. Although he may know that medicine is an art with a scientific basis and may recognise public expectations of medicine to be exaggerated, he is sustained by the idea that medicine can be precise and scientific. He may know that the public wants more than technical proficiency and also asks for less specific forms of medical attention involving caring, humanity and wisdom, yet he is likely to take refuge in his purely medical and 'scientific' roles. He feels justified in bringing moral weight and even coercion to bear on the patient and relatives because he 'knows what is good for them', and he interprets this as giving them an extended and/or more comfortable life.

A doctor, when deciding to press for a particular line of management, will consider his own feelings—imagining himself in the position of a patient left, for example, with some defect unremedied. He will judge the expected quality of life resulting from the procedure to be adopted, or not adopted, according to his own experience and enjoyment of life. These experiences are frequently quite different from the experiences of his patients.

The risk is that the effect on the individual doctor of large numbers of people and institutions seeking and accepting his judgments must be to raise within him self-images which are larger than life. The longer he has been in the practice of medicine the more he feels justified in extending the scope of his 'art', especially when as an ageing doctor he realises that his grip on the scientific element in his work is slackening. As medicine becomes less a solitary and 'horse and buggy' activity it becomes more dependent on other professions and larger and larger machines. This may strengthen his confidence in his authority to make life and death decisions, but it may also encourage him to extend his practice beyond what he is certain he knows.

However, medicine shares the increasing complexity of life and the increasing necessity to accept the say-so of the 'expert', whether he is a doctor or a plumber. The doctor as one expert among others feels, at one level, that the exercise of his skill needs no more justification than that of other experts who just as clearly influence the daily lives and futures of the population, e.g. engine drivers, power workers or dustmen. But death limits his expertise and authority, and demands re-examination of many of his cherished assumptions.

An attempt to define 'Pre-death', by a District Nurse

Pre-death is the complex situation in which it becomes obvious from changes that are occurring, that the patient is appealing for help, for proper management and care, aware that he/she is 'going downhill'. Medical diagnosis and prognosis are not sufficient to define the pre-death phase, but rather it is necessary to take account of the very definite changes in the patient's behaviour (Isaacs: *The Concept of Pre-Death*, 1971)

There is an identifiable point in which a) the patient's behaviour changes with the realisation of the onset of death; b) the staff's behaviour changes in relation to and in interaction with the patient; c) relatives' behaviour changes subtly, often unconsciously, in relation to the dying patient, due to cues from both patient and staff. There emerges a new inter-personal phase, that of *pre-death*, which it is important to recognise and identify for proper management and care of the dying. The appropriate preparation of relatives also depends upon it. There is a definite stage at which medical and nursing staff need to face and accept their failure to effect a cure and to accept that a shift to a more caring type of management is necessary. (Cf. Cartwright, A. et al, 1973; Glaser, B. and Strauss, A. L., 1965).

The only possible confirmation of a correct diagnosis of the pre-death phase is subsequent death, and even then it is possible that pre-death and dying have not been clearly distinguished. Notwithstanding the difficulties, it is of professional and ethical importance to attempt a reliable assessment or diagnosis of pre-death, as its management in terms of intervention should be specific to it in the same way as the management of appendicitis is specific to the condition.

Patient's cues. The patient's cues provide the commonality in the assessment, and stimulate the search for observable and/or definable features. The identifiable pre-death period—as opposed to actually dying—is absent when the patient is unaware of approaching death. It is absent because its identification is dependent on patient cues. Therefore, recognition of the pre-death stage places an immediate ethical responsibility on professionals and other caring persons. The patient's cues are his acknowledgment of his condition with its inherent expectation of appropriate management. On the basis of experience, the non-verbal cues are most often changes in behaviour; therefore, specific to and dependent on the patient's normal behaviour.

Tentative definition. A person can be taken to have entered the pre-death state if: (i) He is suffering from a (diagnosed) condition which has a fatal prognosis; (ii) His condition is deteriorating in spite of medical treatment; (iii) He is deviating markedly from his normal behaviour, e.g. depressed/elated, quiet/garrulous, pleasant/aggressive, placid/anxious; (iv) Ceases to take an active part/interest in his treatment or other aspects of his care, such as food, diversional activity, etc.; (v) May in addition express explicitly his awareness of dying.

In general practice most deaths are sudden and therefore there can be no clear 'pre-death' phase or planning of terminal care. However, to talk about pre-death is to talk about the kind of situations where there is time to mount a team approach, where there is opportunity to put into practice some of the ideals of good terminal care. The attempt to provide a functional definition of pre-death has general value insofar as it represents an attempt to review the different kinds of response and approach to patient management which different terminal situations demand, an opportunity for reflection on professional attitudes to death and bereavement, and to identify the moral responsibilities and dilemmas which professionals face in terminal care.

Discussion and identification of four problems

The Physician's account of the basis of the doctor's self-justification for becoming involved in terminal care illustrates that medical and technical grounds, while they may be the most important reasons for the doctor's intervention, are not in principle or in practice sufficient. Value-judgments have to be made by the doctor, just as the hopes and expectations of the patient are based on certain assumptions about the trustworthiness of doctors and the value of health-care. The doctor's ability to make these difficult moral judgments, and his confidence in performing his task, including riskful procedures, is based not only on his training, knowledge and experience, but belief in the value of the service he performs for suffering humanity, of the pursuit of scientific medicine, and of his personal and professional integrity.

The District Nurse's attempt to define 'Pre-Death' also illustrates that it is not purely a functional problem or technical issue, for it raises immediately questions about what constitutes good professional management of the dying, and what constitutes a good death for the patient and relatives. The difficulty and ambiguity of any definition of 'Pre-Death'—depending as it does on the sensitive perception of many related attitudes and behaviours—illustrates once again that value-judgments have to be made which determine the nature and direction of terminal care. These relate in particular to the ideals governing doctor-patient or nurse-patient communication and the question of how to secure good understanding and cooperation between the members of the Primary Medical Care Team (PMCT) or the Ward Team.

In both cases the central moral issues in professional practice emerged as concerned with the value assumptions built in to the attempt to define the problems of terminal care as questions of professional management, and the assumptions underlying talk about the need for better inter-professional communication in the care of the dying and the bereaved.

The following problem-areas were identified in discussion:

(i) The ambiguities introduced into the 'contract' with the patient by the recognition that the patient has entered the 'Pre-Death' phase.

(ii) The tension on the health-care team created by the conflicting demands for inter-professional cooperation and consultation on the one hand, and the demand for someone to exercise authority and take decisions, on the other.

(iii) The dilemmas faced by the professional where conflicts arise between his general professional responsibilities including his duties to other patients and the exceptional demands of the dying patient.

(iv) The tendency of the professional to use the technique of definition as a device to solve moral dilemmas, by re-defining the issue as a 'problem' which is susceptible to management in terms of familiar knowledge and techniques, rather than to confront the moral issues involved and seek some courageous solution to them.

(i) *'Contracts' with the dying.* The circumstances in which the patient approaches the doctor and requests help—'under the duress of fear and need'—create the framework of obligations and responses which tend to determine the relationship. The dialectic of Authority and Dependence, Expertise and Need, Responsibility and Compliance, Confidence and Trust which are implicit in the doctor-patient relationship show that from the outset the relationship is both clinical and moral. The doctor never acts in a therapeutic situation which is free of moral assumptions, but in the confidence that what he does is 'right' both in the sense of medically correct and in the sense of being in the best interests of the patient. Knowing 'what is in the best interests of the patient' not only means responding sensitively to the interests and needs of the individual, but implicitly involves general convictions about what is good and desirable for human beings. Thus the self-confidence which the doctor requires in order to act decisively is not only dependent on his medical training and experience, but crucially upon the trust which the patient has in him. One of the reasons why confidentiality is so important in the doctor-patient relationship is that patient trust and medical confidence both relate to it in a fundamental way. In sharing confidences with the doctor the patient exposes his vulnerability and expresses his confidence in the doctor. In respecting those confidences the doctor acknowledges the fact that he depends on the patient's trust for the right, confidence and authority to act. It is this confidential relationship which is put under strain when the doctor realises that the patient is dying. He may feel unable to communicate this fact to the dying patient and his own confidence and authority to act may be undermined.

In general there are important differences between the circumstances where the patient is able to approach the doctor himself, and where the patient is *non compos mentis*. Both are governed by the same value assumptions and moral obligations. So long as the patient is able to communicate with and negotiate with the doctor he can be said to authorise the doctor's various interventions—however artificial this may appear in the light of the patient's actual circumstances. Once the patient is no longer capable of authorising the doctor's actions, the 'contract' does not cease to operate. On the contrary, the doctor acquires a double responsibility to safeguard the patient's interests to the best of his ability. The legitimacy of the doctor's actions has to be seen partly in terms of fidelity to the intentions of the original contract, and partly to the standards of integrity and proficiency proper to his profession. If it is still possible to communicate with the patient who has been diagnosed as dying, this may create a painful dilemma for the doctor—as to whether he should communicate his prognosis to the patient in the interests of fidelity to the confidential nature of his contract with the patient, and in the interests of obtaining informed consent for whatever procedures are adopted or stopped.

In practice the informality of the doctor-patient 'contract' leaves many issues unspecified and unclear. This may often be in the best interests of both parties, for it does not over-commit the patient and allows a wide discretion to the doctor. Such 'contracts' are not normally open to re-negotiation as things go along. In practice they tend to be governed by all sorts of inhibitions and unspoken assumptions. The pattern of a relationship once established tends to persist in the same form and neither doctor nor patient are likely to initiate changes in the relationship.

Prognosis may be an anxiously uncertain art, but the fact remains that when the diagnosis of a fatal condition is reached, and more particularly when the patient becomes aware that his condition is terminal, a new state arises which changes the basis of the relationship between doctor and patient. The assumptions of therapeutic optimism underlying the ordinary 'contract' are profoundly modified. The patient's right to know, which underlies the confidential and therapeutic relationship, acquires a new meaning in the face of imminent death, and the patient's right to self-determination acquires a new poignancy. These factors modify the terms on which the relationship between doctor and patient may be conducted in the terminal phase. Telling the truth may entail the re-negotiation of these informal 'contracts' as the doctor has to admit his helplessness and inability to cure, or as the patient contracts out by deciding to go home to die; as the doctor offers care and support and fidelity to the end and the patient accepts that he has to settle for comfort. The unwillingness to discuss bad prognoses with patients may be due to the general uncertainty of the situation, but it may also relate in part to unwillingness to re-examine and re-negotiate the basis of the 'contract' between doctor and patient.

(ii) *Tension on the inter-professional team*. The value of an inter-professional team approach to terminal care has been greatly emphasised in recent times. However, the problems and difficulties have not been discussed sufficiently frankly or critically—particularly the problems of joint decision-making. The benefits of the team approach are not unambiguous. On the one hand the co-ordination of efforts and resources can have great benefit for patient care, and team co-operation can provide useful mutual support for members of the professional team. On the other hand having more people around on the team does not necessarily increase the

9

confidence of individual professionals, ⌈subjected to the⌉ critical scrutiny of other experts; it can lead to delay in reaching crucial decisions, to the abrogation of responsibility and conflict where there is no agreement as to who should accept authority for difficult moral decisions; it can underline the charismatic relationship of the individual doctor, nurse or other professional where the importance of particular relationships to individual patients is not appreciated.

Several problems militate against team management becoming a panacea. Healing has been traditionally associated with the power, skill and influence of the individual 'healer' and it is doubtful whether there can be healing in this sense in a team. The move towards group-practice and the shift-working hospital doctor assumes that medical problems are reducible to problems of technical management and ignores the therapeutic importance of continuity of care in meaningful personal relationships. Secondly, in reality the problems of patient-care vary from the acute medical ward to psychiatry, from clinical surgery to the care of the elderly and the dying. Each requires a different solution in terms of team organisation and patient management. In general the acute state requires a more hierarchical, authoritarian and doctor-centred form of organisation. Psychiatry, geriatric medicine and terminal care allow a more democratic form of inter-professional co-operation. Thirdly, the realities of varying degrees of training, experience and skill mean that a completely egalitarian model of team organisation is unlikely to work in practice. For example, the fact that the majority of nurses are unqualified, or that the inexperienced houseman has to rely on the experienced ward sister, militates against simple equality on the team. Further, differing kinds of skill and expertise of different professionals may have different importance or significance depending on the kind of decision to be taken by the team. Finally, patients may prefer to choose their own doctor or particular health-care professional as their confidant and may resent management by a more impersonal team. Consumer resistance may dictate that health-services develop a less managerial and more patient-orientated pattern of health-care. (Cartwright, A., *Patients and their Doctors*, 1967)

(iii) *The cure or care dilemmas.* The professional role of the doctor, and to some extent of the nurse, is predicated upon certain assumptions about medicine as a healing art. The priority given to life-saving cure-orientated medicine in professional training, in the expectations of the public, and in the practical allocation of health-care resources, has a profound effect on the attitudes of practising professionals, determining their priorities in patient care. In spite

10

of official pronouncements about the economic priority to be given to the low-prestige 'caring' areas of medicine, of mental and physical handicap, geriatric medicine and mental illness, the balance of priorities in medicine in general is unlikely to change much. The fairly recent epidemiological changes in the pattern of morbidity and mortality in modern society may gradually affect the way that doctors and nurses are taught and their consequent attitudes; but the cure-dominated values are likely to persist so long as there is a hope that science and new techniques may discover ways of effecting cures for human ills and so long as medicine continues to be seen as a healing art.

These values are translated into more specific obligations in terms of the rules of conduct applicable to the exercise of the professional's role. What is 'right' or 'wrong' is defined for him by: a) the rules of professional etiquette, b) the tradition and 'case law' of medical ethics, and c) the limits of social morality. The rules of professional etiquette,created and perpetuated by a doctor's professional peers, powerfully affect the style in which he performs his functions and the limits within which he ordinarily acts. The accepted 'house style' on a particular ward or in a particular medical unit, for example, will define the form and limits within which doctors and other staff express their curing and caring roles. The ethico-legal considerations, defined by rule and precedent, which comprise medical ethics in the technical sense, define by exclusion of the worst what it is permissible or impermissible for health-care staff to do. Finally the rules and demands of social morality may on the one hand inhibit the doctor from performing certain acts which are socially unacceptable, e.g. euthanasia or termination of pregnancy, even if he personally believes it is morally justified, but they may also encourage him to act 'over and above the call of duty' insofar as he recognises social and moral responsibilities transcending the narrower requirements of his professional duty.

The situation of the dying patient challenges the priorities and values of ordinary medical practice. Whether or not doctors and other staff should 'strive officiously to keep alive' relates to fundamental questions about what is ultimately desirable and good for man—to survive as long as possible or to die a good death. But besides these general moral questions terminal care faces the health-care professional with other more specific questions about the nature and limits of his professional role. To choose to work with the dying may thus be personally difficult and demanding, but it may also require a reversal of the ordinary professional priorities.

11

(iv) *Definition and the justification of professional intervention in terminal care*. Justification of professional intervention in terminal care, and the solution of the practical and moral difficulties associated with the care of the dying and the bereaved depends to some extent on how the problems are defined. Definition is an important tool of the professional in deciding how 'problems' are to be 'solved'. The physician's attempt to define the basis of the doctor's right to intervene in terminal care, and the district nurse's attempt to define Pre-Death, are examples of professionals employing the techniques of definition to clarify the nature of the problems, to justify professional intervention, to distinguish the different roles of doctors, nurses and other caring persons, and to decide on the best course of patient management. (Cf. Clarke, D. D. and Clarke, D. M. 1977) If there is, for example, a real moral dilemma about the administration of pain-killing drugs to the dying patient, because they may shorten his life, then this kind of problem is not solved by acquiring more medical information or by the refinement of techniques for the administration of drugs, but by the courage to confront the fact that a value judgment has to be made. Someone has to decide that it is better that the patient should die sooner but in comfort, or that the patient ought to be kept alive as long as possible, even if in pain. To engage in philosophical argument about the definition of rights and responsibilities may be necessary to clarify the theoretical issues involved, but to do so in an urgent practical situation would be irresponsible and a device to escape making ethical choices. To seek to redefine a moral dilemma as a practical 'problem' can also be a means to avoid accepting the moral responsibility which making value-judgments and ethical decisions implies.

SUGGESTED READING FOR CHAPTER ONE

The studies listed in the Bibliography under Aries (1976), Balint (1957), Boyd (1977), Brauer (1965), Cartwright (1967), Cartwright et al (1973), Choron (1973), Clarke (1977), Cronin (1939), Ferris (1965, 1967), Glaser & Strauss (1965), Gorer (1965), Isaacs (1971), Magee (1977), Saunders (1969).

TWO

Death and Professional Responsibility

DEATH means different things to the doctor, the nursing staff, the chaplain, the relatives and the others involved. The way each regards death has to do with the part they play in the event. The way the professionals involved define death is directly related to the responsibilities which they exercise, to the functions which they perform. In the last chapter we saw that definition is a tool which we use to organise reality both theoretically and practically, and the significance of definitions has to be seen in their relation to human intentions and activities, in their relation to the different roles and functions, rights and responsibilities exercised by individuals.

For example, the decision that death has occurred is and traditionally has been a medical responsibility. The doctor has the responsibility to decide, on the best available scientific grounds, what constitute adequate theoretical and practical criteria for the determination of death. The clinical definition of death may, in a sense, be treated as morally neutral, but its significance cannot be understood apart from the doctor's function, that is, to be society's appointed authority to decide such matters. The activity of defining death cannot be separated entirely from the practical function of the doctor in determining whether death has occurred in a particular case and his responsibility to sign the death-certificate.

On the surface, definitions may appear to be morally neutral, but when we consider their purpose or function in relation to human activity we cannot ignore their moral implications and significance. Certifying a death may not appear to raise moral issues in the case of 'death from natural causes', but they can be seen to be implied—even if only because the doctor's authority, competence and integrity are at stake. However, where there is a 'suspicion of foul play' the nature of the doctor's moral responsibility becomes much more obvious, as it does too where the circumstances of a death are unusual. In relation to current debate about 'brain death' it is obvious that the medical profession has been provoked into a profound re-examination of the traditional

C   13

criteria for determining death, less by the expansion of knowledge than the expansion of the doctor's legal and moral responsibilities —particularly in relation to the termination of life artificially maintained on life-support systems, and in relation to the problems of organ transplantation. The need to protect himself from criticism and litigation drives the professional to seek clarification of the nature and scope of his moral responsibilities, rather than some theoretical interest in medical ethics. In a recent circular to doctors from the Chief Medical Officer for Scotland, on the subject of Brain Death, it is emphasised that doctors' motives for certifying death must be above suspicion:

The conclusion that respiration and a beating heart are being maintained solely by mechanical means and that brain death has occurred, *must, of course, be reached independently of any transplant considerations.* (SHHD/CAMO(78)/.9.1.1978)

The responsibility which the doctor exercises in defining the criteria by which death can be determined, and then applying these criteria in practice, is not some purely scientific and theoretical activity, but a complex practical and moral function which he performs on behalf of society and ultimately in the best interests, in the service, of his patients.

Similarly, the way nurses, chaplains and others view death, define death, has to be interpreted in relation to the way they conceive their roles, and the responsibilities which they exercise. The death of a human being is not a morally neutral event—either for the deceased or for those around him. What his death signifies, whether it is seen as a 'good' or a 'bad' death, relates to what happened in the particular case in question and to the part each has played in the event.

In this chapter we seek to illustrate these general observations by an analysis of contributions by a Surgeon, a Ward Sister and a Chaplain to a symposium on Death and Dying. We are less concerned with the definition of death in the abstract than with what constitutes a 'good death' for the patient and for the professionals involved.

The first contribution, which was presented in February 1976, eight months before the statement of the Conference of Medical Royal Colleges on the Diagnosis of Brain Death (BMJ, 13 Nov. 1976), explores the need for a new definition of death, particularly in terms of the definition of brain death.

A definition of death, by a Surgeon

Until recently, the classical medical definition of death, 'complete and persistent cessation of respiration and circulation' has sufficed. Now, this definition is inadequate, firstly because the widespread use of strong hypnotic and tranquilising drugs produce states where it becomes extremely difficult to tell whether respiration and circulation have ceased; secondly, because of the development of advanced resuscitative techniques by which circulation and respiration may be maintained artificially by machine; and thirdly, because of the needs for living organs for transplantation. Death can be defined as the irreversible loss of living matter. A distinction is made between the properties of the whole person and those of his parts. Thus, extinction of a) personality and of vital functions constitute 'somatic death' and b) of the body tissues; 'molecular' or 'cellular death'. The relevance of these definitions is clear from knowledge that following cessation of circulation, the brain dies in five minutes, the kidneys in one hour, muscle in several hours and skin and nail in several days.

Traditional Signs of Death. The decision that one is dead is medical. The traditional signs are: 1) Cessation of heart beat, detected by listening over the heart for 5 minutes, or if in doubt, by an electrocardiogram; 2) Cessation of respiration confirmed by observation for chest movements over a ten-minute period; 3) Paleness of the skin. 4) Eye signs: i. Absence of corneal and light reflexes. These are the blink when the cornea is touched, contraction of the pupil when a light is shone into it; ii. clouding of the cornea, the eyes assuming a glazed appearance; iii. 'tache noir de la sclerotique', round or oval spots initially on the outer side of the globe, yellowish becoming brown and then black; iv. reduction in intraocular tension; the eyeball becomes soft; v. fragmentation and stasis of the blood in the retinal blood vessels seen through an ophthalmoscope. The blood stream becomes irregular and lumpy. 'Rail-roading' or 'cattle trucking' is caused by clumps of blood cells. 5) Certain other changes that take place after death. These are: i. cooling of the body. Some advise rectal temperature of less than 23.9°C (75°F) as a necessary criterion of death; ii. post-mortem lividity; due to engorgement of the dependent capillary blood vessels by gravitation of blood. The dependent parts of the body other than those exposed to pressure become red in colour; iii. softening of the limbs, the muscles and skin losing their elasticity and tone. Flattening of contact points occurs. After 2–3 hours rigor mortis develops, the muscles becoming rigid. This starts in the muscles of eyelids and lower jaw and then progressively develops in the muscles of neck, face, chest, upper limbs, trunk, and lower limbs. It usually passes off in 36 hours or longer in a cold environment.

15

Brain Death. The problem of death defined in this way is that it fails to take into account the fact that irreversible brain damage can occur while the circulation and respiration are maintained. This state may be found in patients with severe head injuries but is most commonly seen in those who are maintained on a respirator.

The definition of brain death is not easy. In France, clinical death is considered to have taken place when a person is affected by lesions incompatible with life though maintained in a state of vegetable existence by various devices and when an electroencephalogram has shown for a period of at least ten minutes lack of function from higher nervous centres; that is to say, when the EEG tracing is a straight line.

In Germany, 'if the patient is unconscious for at least 12 hours, and if spontaneous respiration ceases, bilateral mydriasis (dilatation of the pupil) sets in, the pupils do not react to light, reflexes are extinct and the EEG tracing shows an iso-electric line for at least one hour without interruption, then the patient can be considered dead, notwithstanding the fact that the heart may still respond to artificial stimulation'.

Both introduce the electrical activity of the brain (EEG recording) as a sign of death, but it is not clear how many sites of the brain must be monitored or how long this should be for. In 1968, 24 hours of flat EEG recordings was regarded as death; it has now been reduced to one hour. Conversely, there is recent evidence that EEG recordings of continued cerebral activity may sometimes be associated with other clinical evidence of irrecoverable brain damage.

The codes developed in Minnesota and in New York now fall back on using circulatory and respiratory sites to determine when structural brain damage is irreversible. Before accepting the patient as dead, it must be shown that spontaneous breathing will not occur during a three-minute period of disconnection from the respirator, while oxygen is delivered to the patient in a standard way. This is repeated each 12 hours.

There must, of course, also be evidence of severe structural brain damage; absence of all brain stem reflexes, fixed pupils, absent corneal reflexes, and no motor responses.

Conclusions. It seems reasonable to suggest that a patient is dead when he lapses into final unconsciousness and out of communication with other human beings. Perhaps the only 'good death' is therefore sudden loss of consciousness which is irreversible in a patient who otherwise was fit and had no premonition or warning of what was to occur.

16

The surgeon's contribution was criticised by the Group in so far as it tended to represent the doctor's functions in defining/determining death as purely technical. It obscured two facts, first that the circumstances in which the doctor exercises his responsibilities have changed with the advent of organ and tissue transplants, and second that it is chiefly anxiety about the extent and nature of these new responsibilities that has provoked attempts at a new definition of death in terms of brain death.

The advice of the Chief Medical Officer of the SHHD was seen to be unrealistic for it was maintained that it is impossible in practice for decisions about the termination of life-support to be made completely 'independently of any transplant considerations'. It was argued that what the doctor is actually doing when he certifies death has subtly changed with the possibility that some of the organs of his patient may be used to help another patient or patients. Previously the doctor was only concerned with the deceased, his ex-patient, when he certified death. Now the certification of death takes into consideration other patients' interests. The interests of other mortally ill patients may well have to be considered when determining the precise moment that life-support systems are switched off.

The anxiety aroused by the need for the doctor to exercise these additional moral responsibilities in defining death was, it was claimed, the chief reason why there was a feeling of urgency about the need for a satisfactory definition of brain death. It was felt that there ought to be more candidness about the extent and nature of anxiety felt in this area, first so that the moral issues involved could be confronted and frankly discussed both within the medical profession and with the concerned public, and secondly so that thought might be given to how intra-professional and inter-professional support could be given to doctors faced with difficult moral dilemmas.

The surgeon's view that 'perhaps the only "good death" is therefore sudden loss of consciousness which is irreversible', was criticised on the grounds that it tends to view the problem too narrowly from what the doctor imagines is the patient's point of view. It was questioned whether the doctor, concerned with the alleviation of suffering, does not tend to view the most desirable thing for the patient as the alleviation of suffering; whether it might not possibly be desirable for the dying patient to have time to come to terms with the fact, and it was pointed out that sudden death could often be traumatic for the relatives, causing complications in bereavement. The question of what constitutes a good

17

death, it was suggested, cannot be adequately answered by considering the dying patient in isolation.

Varieties of death on the ward, by a Ward Sister

For nurses, the definition of death is simple—it is when the doctor says the patient is dead. However, that leads immediately to a possible moral dilemma: What happens when a doctor is not available (e.g. all in theatre)? Does the nurse tell the relative or not?

I cannot think of death as a separate issue on its own. It is the end of something which occurs in a hospital context. You remember the person, the illness, the events surrounding it, the people involved, but you don't recall the death as such.

The 'variety' and 'types' of death: (i) The 'unconscious death', e.g. post-operative death in neurosurgery—when the patient does not regain consciousness and dies. Here the needs of the relatives and the nurses are important. You know the patient is going to die, but sometimes they take an unconscionably long time to do so. This may be a good death for the patient, but not for the nurses or relatives. The doctor can withdraw, but the nurses often feel isolated and have to cope with the anxious and distressed relatives.

(ii) The 'abrupt' death, e.g. death following head injury, cerebral haemorrhage, heart attack—the sudden death which comes unexpectedly and unprepared. Sometimes it happens that a patient in for a minor complaint dies suddenly. You are all unprepared for it—the medical staff, nursing staff and relatives. There may be a sense of shock around compounded by a feeling of guilt that something has been overlooked. You have had no time to build up a relationship with the relatives nor even sometimes with the patient. Communication can be very difficult. You don't know about the patient's relationship with the relatives. You can't say 'He must have been a marvellous man' because he might have been a stinker! You are uncertain how much is known and emotional reactions can be strong—so you withdraw.

(iii) The 'machine' death—where life is maintained only by a machine, in a body which has ceased to function in any way, but the machine will not cease to function until someone turns it off. This is a dangerous area. You give drugs to 'relieve' what you believe may be non-existent pain . . . there is pretended innocence, ignorance, understanding . . . the word 'euthanasia' is not used. However we all function within this conspiracy. Is it necessary? All nurses must know that they have contributed to euthanasia—you give drugs 'to kill the pain' and an hour later the patient dies. The relatives say to the doctor or ward-staff 'We hope he won't suffer for long' or 'We hope he doesn't linger unduly'. There are complex undercurrents of feeling in such situations and great tensions in the exercise of your responsibilities.

(iv) The 'bad' death—this is the death which is painful and/or traumatic for the patient and the nursing staff, where there is mis-handling of the death, the patient, or the relatives. The bad death is always remembered. For example a death in the middle of the ward at visiting time is a messy unpleasant death for all involved. You try to resuscitate the patient, you fail. There is misunderstanding, distress, it leaves a bad taste in the mouth. Another example is the patient who dies fully aware of what is happening. It might take only minutes, but it is a long time for those concerned. Such deaths may be distressing for the patient and disturbing for the nursing staff because they can't help feeling they have failed somehow.

Should you talk to student nurses about such deaths? Or will talking to them about such issues only make them more frightened? It needs a lot of self-awareness and confidence to talk about deaths on the ward, or to suggest that the subject is discussed. You cannot avoid the problems in nursing and we have to learn to face the fact that there are sometimes situations where there is no way that they can be handled well. Talking these things out together, sharing the guilt and anxiety, can be a great comfort and support.

The death of a child. There are no 'good' deaths among children. Death is indecent. The only acceptable deaths are the deaths of unaware (neurosurgical) patients. The chronically ill child knows when he is dying. He withdraws from the hospital staff. Death of a child rarely brings parents together. More often they are left incapable of helping each other, incapable of even touching each other. There is a sense of failure at the death of a child. Unhelpful relatives may arrive unhelpfully from Australia. And there is nothing about all this in the procedure manual. Often it is only experience of such situations that can help you learn how to deal with them.

The 'communication' of death. How do you tell the relatives? Do you use the word 'dead' or 'died', or fall back on euphemisms? A large number of nurses, asked these questions, replied that they would say 'Betty has died . . .' However they were also quite sure that someone else (the doctor) would actually tell the relatives!

But who should tell them? It is usually the doctor. But what happens when he is a locum or it is this first day on the ward? Is the doctor always the 'right' person or the 'best' person? Or just the 'expected' person? This should be a matter of flexibility and willingness to recognise who is the most appropriate person —in terms of who has had the most contact with the patient/ family. Often it is the Ward Sister who should do it.

Should the information be given by telephone? Is it humane to say 'the patient's condition has deteriorated—come quickly' when in fact death has already occurred? The relatives may be subjected to a journey of anxiety because you feel it is kinder. However, to tell the truth outright can be a bad experience. You don't know the circumstances 'at the other end of the line'. What happens if you break the news and there is just silence at the other end? (These issues were a matter of concern to Widows and Members of CRUSE as well as the Police—see Appendices at the end of the Report.)

The effect of death in the ward. Nurses in an acute ward tend to feel that death is 'untidy' and set about clearing it away with indecent haste—'dies, dealt with, goes to the mortuary'. The patient goes in a bizarre vehicle. The screens are drawn and the other patients read the papers. The screens are pulled back. The death bed is already made up and the nurses pretend that nothing has happened. If a patient does express distress at the presence of a dying patient, what do you do? Do you tidy away the dying patient before he is dead—into a side room? Then there are the possessions which have to be tidied away. The saddest thing is the bundle of personal belongings.

To have been at the receiving end, to receive the transparent plastic bag of clothes, etc., is distressing. You do not know what to say. Death is an area where a lot can be done to give nurses better insight, to help make them less afraid. Death in hospital affects and involves a variety of people and it is as well to recognise this and develop the ability to talk about it with openness and truth.

In comparison to the surgeon, the Ward Sister's contribution illustrated in a more obvious way that death is significant as an interpersonal event and that the circumstances which make that event 'good' or 'bad' for those involved are directly related to the way they affect interpersonal relations.

The Ward Sister was particularly concerned with the effect of the patient's death on the relatives and the nursing staff. A 'bad death' in her terms was a death that caused distress to the relatives and directly or indirectly to the ward staff—nurses being particularly distressed if the patient was alert and aware of what was going on. The situations which she described were mainly those in acute medical wards where it would be unlikely that the dying patient would have time to reflect on his dying. By implication a 'good death' was one where the patient was not aware or distressed by dying, and when the medical and nursing staff could feel confident that they had managed well and handled the relatives satisfactorily.

Her suggestion that drugs are sometimes given to relieve non-existent pain was questioned by two different groups of people — first by those who maintained that in general this is not done and anyone who did so would be guilty of malpractice, next by those who argued that more commonly doctors and nurses have a poor record on pain relief and are more likely to under-provide rather than over-provide opiates. Yet others agreed that euthanasia is covertly practised and insisted that the issue ought to be more seriously and honestly discussed.

Different reactions to death and dead bodies were also discussed. Doctors were criticised for their matter-of-fact treatment of patients once they were dead, sometimes showing indifference to the reactions of relatives and others, including nursing staff, whose grief is expressed in terms of attachment to and reverence for the body of the deceased. Nurses were criticised for their anxious haste to remove the body from the ward and to conceal the facts of death from other patients. It is desirable that there should be more openness about death on the ward, that other patients should be encouraged to talk out the anxieties provoked in them by a death on the ward. The example of St Christopher's Hospice was cited — where the curtains are pulled during death, but patients are encouraged to talk about it afterwards — for this makes death a social event in the ward environment as it is in society and helps patients cope with their bereavement at the loss of a fellow patient. The design and environment of large general hospitals makes this kind of openness difficult to achieve, and in any case this kind of approach is not always appropriate, as certain patients did not wish to discuss these matters.

What it means to die, by a Chaplain

The Chaplain is often seen as the harbinger of death — the one who precedes the funeral directors around the wards. This perception is perhaps undesirable from the chaplain's point of view, but not without significance, for the fear of death is a significant factor in patients admitted to hospital and the chaplain may be the one to whom these fears are voiced. A large proportion of people admitted to hospital request a visit from chaplains and there is considerable evidence that this is because they are frightened of dying or want to talk about death and dying.

It is the function of the minister to be available, not to impose himself on the dying. It is questionable whether ministers have the right to be by the bedside of dying patients, unless invited. Their function is to support, to listen, to help patients cope with their feelings and fears. At a deeper level the chaplain is there to help the patient wrestle with the great questions of meaning which arise in death. Specifically 'religious counselling' is most often inappropriate, however willingness to explore the searching metaphysical questions people ask about the meaning of life is certainly part of the chaplain's task. More often it is a matter of helping people work through their complex emotional reactions to death—emotions which include anger, loneliness and isolation, anxiety and guilt or depression. Patients, especially men, fear making a fool of themselves. They may regret lost things, may be anxious regarding their families, their jobs or finance, may grieve over unfinished situations and unresolved relationships.

The supportive role of the chaplain is made more difficult when a patient suspects that he is dying but has not been told, and this problem is worst in units which adopt a policy of secrecy. People have a right to know if they want to know, and no doctor or relative has the right to withhold from patients that they are dying. The more a person feels that he is dying but is surrounded by people who deny this, the greater is the feeling of isolation. People may want to know in order to put their affairs in order, or for more personal reasons. 'Comfort' to the dying in some circumstances may well mean telling them the truth. The chaplain's role may well be to challenge 'the conspiracy of silence'.

Relatives also react to death and the prospect of it in different ways and the chaplain can share the grieving experience, help them to cope and support them during the period of pre-death. Chaplains also have a function in counselling nurses and doctors who are facing death and the dilemmas it brings. Concern with the questions of being and meaning is common to us all, but tends to be evoked in a poignant way by death, not only for the dying patient but for all those around him. The chaplain should represent the possibility that it makes sense to face and explore those questions either alone or with others.

The Chaplain, by contrast with the Surgeon and the Ward Sister, was primarily concerned with the significance of the event for the dying patient himself, and for the grieving relatives. In support of this view Dr Cecily Saunders was quoted as having said: 'When I die I hope it is of cancer—because I believe most of the pain and distress associated with cancer can be controlled with proper medical and nursing care, and besides most patients remain lucid until very near the end. This gives the patients the opportunity to come to terms with their own death and to work out some of the anticipatory grief with their loved ones.'

This view seemed to imply that a good death is a slow death. Many felt that a brief terminal phase was to be preferred as less harrowing to all concerned—to patient, relatives and staff. The view was also expressed that there is a risk that hospice-based death, particularly death from cancer, may become a paradigm of what death is and ought to be like. This would be unhelpful since the majority of deaths are relatively sudden, occur either at home or in general hospitals where the standards of terminal care cannot be so good as they are in specialised units, and also because cancer accounts only for about a fifth of all deaths. The value of hospices as 'centres of excellence' was recognised, but the education of public attitudes to a more realistic understanding of death and dying required a recognition of the epidemiologically typical forms of death and dying rather than the idealised and rather special circumstances seen in hospices.

The chaplain's contribution focuses attention on the kind of patient with whom the chaplain is likely to be involved—the patient who is to some extent in control of the situation, where he knows what is happening, can face and accept his condition and can perhaps be helped to affirm the meaning and value of his life in some kind of recognition that suffering and pleasure are interwoven in human experience. The situation of such a patient makes it possible to discuss the question of what constitutes a good death less in terms of the external circumstances or the standard of medical and nursing care, and more in terms of the patient's capacity to integrate the experience of dying and his perception of himself and of life in general.

The chaplain's view was criticised as failing to emphasise sufficiently that a good death in his terms presupposed that pain, nausea, breathlessness and depression etc. had been sufficiently controlled for the patient to be capable of reflection on his emotional state or on metaphysical questions. It was stressed that in part at least a 'good death' is made possible by good medical and nursing care, and that patient, doctor, nurses, relatives, chaplain and other caring persons are all functionally related in the process of achieving good terminal care.

23

Discussion and identification of problems

The Group identified three major problem areas in relation to the death of the patient: i) The question of the definition of a 'good death' in terms that do justice to the needs of the dying patient, the relatives and the medical and nursing staff, including other caring persons; ii) the question of the rights of the dying patient in relation to how, when and where to die, including problems of voluntary euthanasia and the role of professionals in 'easing the patient's passage towards death'; iii) the question of the relative rights of family members as against those of the dying patient, and the rights and responsibilities of doctors and other health-care professionals in determining the form of terminal care provided.

i) In discussing 'What is a Good Death?' most detailed comment was provided by a Physician and a District Nurse whose views are summarised here. Their personal views were widely endorsed by the Working Group, and also independently by members of CRUSE (Edinburgh Branch), and the group of Widows, Widowers and Bereaved Parents, whose reports are contained in the Appendix.

Physician. We need to distinguish between 'premature' and 'timely' death. Premature death (e.g. in a child) is always regrettable. But when undesirable experience outweighs desirable experience, when the balance of negative input exceeds positive, then death ceases to be premature. Death in the elderly may be timely if the positive balance cannot be restored. For the aged their friends may have 'gone', the world may have changed and become a strange and hostile place. They may indicate their readiness by saying 'It's time to go', 'I've lived long enough'.

It is questionable whether death and suffering are valuable experiences. Pain has no value in prospect, it may have in retrospect. Because pain has no moral value in itself, it cannot be wrong to endeavour to secure its relief, and anxieties about dying patients becoming addicted to habit-forming drugs are beside the point.

A 'good death' is therefore not 'premature'; it is pain free and not associated with protracted loss of functions; it is not public; it is preferably in a familiar place.

The doctor's professional role in relation to the dying patient is not a specialist one, because in most cases the care of the dying is an extension of the previous role of caring for the ill patient. The doctor depends very much at this stage on the co-operation of the nursing staff and the whole team as well as on the relatives. Decisions regarding treatment or termination of treatment are always taken by at least three people—a senior doctor, junior doctor and nurse. Relief of pain must be accompanied by relief of

24

other discomforts (e.g. depression, nausea, dyspnoea). There is a technology and the doctor must know it. If he isn't a good clinical engine then he is nothing at all.

District Nurse. The recognition of terminality is important so that positive care for the dying can follow acceptance of a forthcoming death. A 'good death' presupposes that care is available at the proper time and in an appropriate manner. Dying at home may be desirable in most cases, but too often patients die at home because they have nowhere to go. In the case of long-term illness periods of hospitalisation may be of great benefit to the patient and relief to the family. However, death at home has many advantages and is often the expressed wish of both patients and relatives. Families are usually concerned that their dying relative should have the best care available, and often need reassurance and practical help (e.g. with nursing, laundry service, technical aids, etc.) so that it can be provided at home.

Death in the home differs from death in the hospital. In the hospital the medical and nursing staff control the situation. In the home the patient and the relatives have more say; the doctor adopts a minimal role; the district nurse often develops a close relationship with patient and relatives. (The attachment of the nurse can cause problems if the situation becomes too emotional for her to cope. She may 'withdraw' by not visiting so frequently.)

A 'good death' is free from pain and discomfort. It is a situation where the patient has continuing emotional support. It is a death where the patient retains self-respect and still feels lovable. It is a situation where the patient maintains their individuality.

The nurse's role is to assess the total situation in terms of the help needed, to intervene with nursing help where appropriate, and to co-operate with other professionals in providing required support. The concept of a 'good death' to some extent 'represents' an ideal. In practice many factors may militate against the achievement of the ideal. For example, there may be lack of consensus among the professionals involved about telling the prognosis to the patient and/or relatives, or relatives may oppose vehemently the telling of the patient (perhaps because they can't face them with the knowledge and its implications). There may be conflict between the doctor and nurse about the appropriate level of medication for pain relief. The nurse may herself be afraid, and unable to inspire confidence. The nurse may withdraw and rationalise not visiting. There may be practical difficulties in obtaining an institutional place if and when the relatives can't cope. There may be lack of clarity about what the patient desires, the relatives want and the nurse thinks appropriate.

25

ii) The rights of the dying patient were discussed in a preliminary way. In general it was emphasised that dying is a highly indviduail, lonely and unique experience, and that consequently moral concern for the dying must include allowance for the individual, where possible, to choose the situation and circumstances of his/her death. Where there is no choice possible or where the individual cannot express his will, painful dilemmas arise for relatives and professionals alike. Insufficiently purposeful intervention can lead to inadequate help being given to the patient and family, over-solicitous care can result in unnecessary investigations, over-medication and the prolongation of useless 'half-life'.

From the patient's point of view the initial 'contract' creates three kinds of 'rights'—the right *to privacy*, the right *to know*, and the right *to treatment*. The doctor retains the right to refuse to take on a patient, but once he takes on the patient he has a responsibility to serve the best interests of the patient by respecting these three basic rights. For his part the patient must respect the right of the doctor to diagnose and treat as he thinks appropriate and to be adequately rewarded for his labours—while he as patient retains the right to refuse treatment.

The right to privacy, the right to know and the right to treatment are not unconditional rights and, especially in the context of terminal care, dilemmas arise about how much these rights are subject to qualification in terms of the extraordinary situation of approaching death. The privacy of the dying patient may be sacrificed in last heroic attempts to save his life, confidential information may be passed on to other staff and relatives 'in the best interests of the patient', decisions may be taken to withhold information from the dying patient because 'it might distress him', therapeutic treatment may be terminated as it is decided 'to settle for comfort'.

The relationship between the patient's right to refuse treatment and his 'right' to choose to die was also recognised as an area which is unclear and fraught with uncertainty for health-care staff. Whether the patient has a 'right to voluntary euthanasia', and, whether doctors have a duty to assist in the termination of lives which have become unendurable or vegetative in form, were seen as unresolved dilemmas which arise out of the basic framework of rights and responsibilities which underlie the relationships of patients and doctors to one another, including other health-care staff. These rights issues were seen to require urgently further examination and discussion.

iii) The relative rights of family members as against those of the dying patient, and the extent of the rights and responsibilities of

26

doctors and other health-care professionals to decide on the form of terminal care to be provided, were questions discussed on numerous occasions. They were discussed as questions which not only raise painful dilemmas for individual professionals in particular cases, but also as questions over which there could be strong disagreements between doctors and nurses or between medical staff and social workers or chaplains—as different members of the team defend the interests of different parties, patient or relatives, or as the doctor insists on his responsibility to decide.

The right of the dying patient to choose to die at home, for example, could not be seen as unconditional. While everything possible should be done to assist the family to cope with nursing the dying patient at home and thus enable the wishes of the patient to be respected, it was recognised that in some circumstances where proper patient-care was not possible in the home, or where the health of other family numbers was being put seriously at risk, then the health-care team might have the duty to override the wishes of the dying patient. While it was felt that imminent death does give heightened importance to the rights of the dying patients, because their very lives are at stake, the issue is seldom free of ambiguities in practice—either for the family or for the professionals involved.

These three issues—the definition of 'a good death', the rights of the dying patient, and the rights of other caring persons—were identified as the most important issues relating to death itself, which required further discussion.

SUGGESTED READING FOR CHAPTER TWO

The studies listed in the Bibliography under Becker (1970), Biorck (1967), Conference of Medical Royal Colleges (1976), Forester (1976), Halley (1968), High (1972), Jennet (1975 and 1977), Kennedy (1973), Rachels (1975), Scottish Home and Health Department (1978), Veatch (1972 and 1975).

THREE

Professionals and the Bereaved

THE SERIOUS STUDY of bereavement and the attempt to define the role of different professionals in the support and care of the bereaved is a relatively recent phenomenon. It has generally been assumed that the individual ought to be left to himself to cope with what support he or she can get from family, the community, and perhaps minister or priest. Changing social conditions, in particular greater social mobility, modern housing, and the break-up of the extended family, have made the nuclear family much more vulnerable to distress of crisis proportions when faced with death and bereavement. The tendency for death to be increasingly confined to the elderly means that bereavement is exacerbated for this group by the other problems associated with old age: limited mobility and relative social isolation, increasing physical and mental disability, and difficult physical and economic circumstances. The fact that many widows or bereaved people have no family or community support and lack church connections means that they have to fall back on other professionals for help in times of bereavement. The Social Worker and General Practitioner in particular, as the most readily accessible professionals, tend to be the ones to whom the bereaved turn with their often complex troubles—health problems, financial and housing difficulties, problems of social adjustment and psychological difficulties, as well as the need for simple friendship.

While ministers have traditionally offered consolation and support to the bereaved, it is only recently that other professionals have recognised that they have a positive contribution to make. Ministers have not in the past had any special training or preparation to cope with the problems of bereavement; but increasingly attention is being given to suitable pastoral training for this work. Social Workers, who tend to spend a great deal of time helping people cope with the distress and multiple social and economic difficulties which follow in the wake of death, have, as a relatively new profession, shown considerable interest in the problems of people facing loss of various kinds. The study of bereavement is now built in to many

28

Social Work courses. However, there is still little recognition of the fact that doctors and nurses (other than General Practitioners and District Nurses) have any real responsibilities to the bereaved.

It is not simply when grief manifests itself in bizarre forms or is associated with chronic depression or other 'pathological' symptoms that bereavement ought to be of concern to doctors and nurses. Bereavement is a factor in and function of any relationship with patients when they are dying or with the immediate relatives when death has occurred. When death is sudden there may be special reason for doctor and nurses to be aware of the trauma suffered by relatives and their need for special care and support. Where death is protracted and expected the bereavement suffered by patient and relatives in anticipation of the death should be a matter of concern and attention from the medical and nursing staff. To deny this or to pretend that these are not medical and nursing responsibilities is either to adopt an extremely narrow interpretation of medical care, or to simply attempt to escape from involvement in the emotional stresses and complications of a death.

Since the publication of Freud's *Mourning and Melancholia* (1917) psychiatrists have been interested in the phenomenon of bereavement. However it is much more recently that it has been argued that grief can be viewed as an illness and therefore as in some sense a doctor's responsibility. C. Murray Parkes (1964), for example, argues:

Therapy should, when possible, start before the bereavement and it is not uncommon for a person to get over the worst of his grief before the actual death has occurred. It is important for doctors and relatives of a seriously ill person to see that those most concerned are aware of his approaching death. Too often the true prognosis is kept dark with the object of sparing the feelings of the closest relatives, as a result of which death when it comes is not expected and the shock is great.

His book *Bereavement* (1972) comprises not only a detailed account of the phenomenology of normal and pathological grief, but also a sustained defence of the view that doctors (and nurses) are justified, even obliged, to become involved in the care of the bereaved as an extension of their responsibilities to the dying. Considerable evidence is cited to support the claim that there is an alarming increase in the mortality and morbidity of those suffering bereavement. The doctor's intervention in bereavement is recommended as good preventive medicine as well as a moral responsibility.

Likewise, the more recent study of *Death and the Family*, by Lily Pincus (1976), has focused attention on the effect which patterns of interaction established in a marriage have on the subsequent character of the bereavement. This study has been perceived to be particularly relevant to the work and interests of Social Workers and to thus provide additional justification for their involvement with the bereaved.

The initial involvement of the doctor, nurse, social worker, minister or other caring person with the bereaved tends to follow a direct approach from the bereaved person for help, or to arise naturally out of a relationship which has become established with those concerned during the period of caring for the dying patient. However, specifically professional intervention in the care of the bereaved tends to follow on the explicit *definition* of bereavement as an illness, or as a disturbed psychological state, or as a function of pre-existent patterns of interaction within a marriage, or as a spiritual crisis etc. By defining 'the problem' in terms which fit the knowledge and skills of their profession, each professional group seeks to justify its involvement with the bereaved.

The view that doctors, nurses, social workers and ministers ought to be concerned with the care of the bereaved may be criticised on the grounds that to treat bereavement as an illness is to medicalise the problem, or that to turn it into a psychiatric or social problem is to make the bereaved into dependents, parasitic upon professionals and the social services. Either way value-judgments are built into the definitions from which we argue.

In this chapter we shall first consider two contributions from professionals, each of whom looks at bereavement from the standpoint of their profession. The chaplain is concerned both with the psychological and broader metaphysical significance of bereavement. The Social Worker with bereavement in the context of the individual's capacity to cope with other kinds of loss. Next we consider the reflections on bereavement of four different groups of lay people. The first two (Police and Funeral Directors) could be considered professionals in their own right, but we shall be less concerned with their own contribution to the care of the dying and the bereaved than with their reflections on the performance of other health-care professionals. The second two groups represent in different ways 'the consumer'. CRUSE, the self-help organisation for widows, provides us with some case-based material which illustrates what bereavement means in practice for the bereaved, as well as some recommendations for the improvement of services (see Appendix). A separate group of Widows, Widowers and Bereaved Parents, specially convened to advise the Research Project, also provides some most useful critical feedback on professional services to the dying and the bereaved (see Appendix).

The meaning of bereavement, by a Chaplain

Bereavement means different things to different people and in attempting to describe the circumstances of the bereaved generalisations are inappropriate. Members of the caring professions encounter a wide range of feelings from the shock and numbness of those who have been suddenly and inexplicably bereft to the prolonged emptiness and despair of those who do not ever get over their loss. In between these two extremes we find: denial—'I don't believe it's true'; guilt—'If only I had, or had not . . .'; anger, often expressed against Health Service staff, clergymen, relatives, neighbours and God; doubt and meaninglessness; 'What is there left in life for me?'; an increased sense of responsibility—the widowed father who must face bringing up his children without the shared insights and values of his wife; exhaustion after nursing a sick relative through a terminal illness or visiting repeatedly in hospital over an extended period; the desire to die—'I wish I was with him'; anxiety about the future; loneliness; a keen realisation, perhaps for the first time of how fragile and precarious life is; and depression which is a feature of all grieving and can sometimes attain pathological proportions. The wide range of feelings encountered in the bereaved also include many positive aspects—gratitude for the life of a significant relative or friend often to the point of idealising his character beyond all recognition; gratitude for the care given by professionals, relatives and friends; relief that the pain and distress, the increasing weakness and disability of the dying person has now finally come to an end; faith that the deceased is now with God or has attained that rest and peace which marks the end of life's struggle.

Grief is described by Parkes as 'a process of realisation, the process by which we make real inside us an event which has already occurred outside us'. Grief is recognised as a necessary and healthy response to loss and working through the feelings associated with grieving is an essential part of the adjustment which the bereaved must make if they are to continue with the business of living. There is much truth in the saying attributed to Jesus, 'Happy are those who mourn—for they shall be comforted'. Comfort in bereavement and happiness are more likely to come to those who grieve rather than to those who fail to grieve.

Support for the bereaved comes from a variety of groups and individuals:

a) *The Family*. The sharing of the experience of bereavement within the family is an important means of grieving. Recollections

31

are often shared, confessions made, tensions relieved, reconciliations effected and affirmation given through intimate, loving and trusting relationships. It should also be noted, however, that relationships within the family can be such that tensions are heightened and conflict deepened, even to the point of estrangement when someone who has helped to keep a family together dies.

b) *Friends and Neighbours.* At a practical level this assistance involves visits to the undertaker, the registrar or the local clergyman, but at a much deeper level neighbours and friends can help the bereaved person to cope with loneliness, dependency and the search for meaning.

c) *Doctors and Nurses.* The involvement of Health Service professionals in the care of the bereaved is assuming ever-growing proportions. The way in which the death of a relative is communicated by a doctor and the way in which relatives are handled by the nursing staff in a hospital ward are remembered and often spoken about long afterwards by the bereaved. More and more bereaved people it seems are turning to the medical profession for support. 'Getting something from the doctor' is urged upon the bereaved by their relatives and friends should they be unduly upset and some doctors make a point of visiting the bereaved as a matter of routine and leaving the Valium tablets on the mantelpiece.

It is now well established that bereavement and loss make us illness-prone and that the health of the bereaved is at risk. For that reason community nurses and health visitors, as well as their medical colleagues, have an important function in caring for the bereaved.

d) *Religious Ministry.* The majority of people call on the services of a minister to officiate at a funeral, but even where they do not, the funeral has an important place in the rituals of mourning. It is a public act involving awareness of the inevitability of death, respect for the deceased, and goodwill and concern for the bereaved. At a funeral, beliefs, feelings, attitudes and values about life and death are articulated and shared. The minister's knowledge of the family and of the deceased person can serve to make the funeral service relevant and personal. One of the consequences of the continuing drift of the population away from the church is that at a time of bereavement many families have no relationship of this kind.

Gorer (1965) has shown that about half of the population do not believe in life after death and of the other half who do, their belief takes a large variety of forms. Nevertheless, in bereavement, those who are 'pagan by conviction' still face imponderable questions about the meaning of life and death, and search for answers which are acceptable to them.

After the funeral, ministers can and often do continue to give pastoral support by being the kind of listener who makes it possible for the bereaved to articulate even the most painful, personal feelings, and by expressing in a representative way the care and concern for the bereaved family on the part of others in the local church and community.

e) *Social Work*. Their knowledge and access to the resources in society which are available to assist the bereaved and their families is an especially important factor.

f) *Voluntary Groups*. There are several voluntary organisations which are available to help those who are bereaved. In one way these societies offer a simple extension of the sharing which is essential to mourning. In another way they bring together those who have experienced bereavement themselves and thus afford the bereaved person new insight and understanding of his experience, as well as a valuable opportunity of sharing it.

g) *The dying person*. Finally, support for the bereaved often comes from the dying person himself, especially if he has faced death openly and shared his thoughts about the future with those who are closest to him. Many a widow is sustained in bereavement through something that her late husband said before he died.

Involvement in helping the bereaved can often be painful and time-consuming. In facing the death of others one is made aware of one's own death. In helping those who have experienced loss one is brought up against the possibilities of loss which one faces oneself and one's own ability or inability to cope. Bereaved people above all need time. It is easy to write a prescription or say a prayer or make a phone call to the Department of Health and Social Security. It is much more difficult to understand and help another human being.

Notes on loss and bereavement, by a Social Worker

Loss is a common denominator in many critical situations in life and helping people to face various kinds of loss is part of the routine work and experience of a social worker. Bereavement is a special kind of loss. Understanding bereavement and being able to help others to cope with grief and loss requires that we first examine how we cope with loss ourselves, how we learn to face these situations and integrate them into our experience. If we can achieve a personal understanding of loss we may have something worthwhile to share. Whether or not we will one day be able to train people to cope better with loss, whether or not people can be prepared to face bereavement, this exercise in self-understanding is essential if we are to empathise with the bereaved. The knowledge may not be directly transferable, but it can make for more meaningful identification with others, painful though that may be. The study of death and bereavement can be useful only if it enlarges our understanding and improves our standards of care. If it becomes a theoretical exercise, a means of parcelling up the pain of dealing with people in distress, then we are in danger of abandoning the concept of care in our institutions.

Theoretical understanding of the process of mourning may be helpful as a backcloth, but let us beware of applying standardised remedies to standardised bereavement situations. Perhaps doctors tend to do this—geared as they are to the provision of treatment! The chaplain has described the range of conflictful emotions which may be present in bereavement, and the professional has the responsibility to identify the predominant mood of the bereaved person before intervening—otherwise the form of intervention may be wholly inappropriate. We have to respond to each situation on its own terms, and if we are responding as individuals, if we are sharing our own experiences, then let us make that explicit. How often do we ascribe feelings to people which in fact reflect our own responses to loss or bereavement?

There is a place for better education or preparation for essential life tasks. Many people are woefully ignorant or only vaguely aware of the mechanics of death, burial, benefits, etc. At a time when they are overwhelmed by personal loss they are further undermined by lack of essential practical knowledge and information. Funeral Directors play an important role here as 'managers' of death in our society. Could people not be better informed and in this way prepared for death? A particular message which needs to be impressed on those facing loss and bereavement is: avoid making hasty, irreversible decisions. Social Workers spend a lot of time trying to undo the harm done by those who have acted precipitately in times of stress and bereavement.

It is in the face of abnormal grief that we feel powerless as professionals. How do we cope with the person 'fixed' in bitterness, anger, despair, who makes apparently unrelenting demands on relatives and on the caring professions in the community? Is it not the case that in dealing with such individuals professional boundaries become protective devices? Do we not project the anger, frustration and sense of impotence which such patients/

clients arouse in us on to other professional groups who 'fail to do something'? Social Workers find that doctors frequently label such people as 'social problems', send them round to us and then get upset if they return! We tend to pass such people on rather than share the responsibility. We need to accept that we are making scapegoats of them and should accept our corporate responsibility to help them. Social Workers have only themselves to blame in many instances for failing to be explicit about what they can and cannot do and for setting themselves up as the carers—or indeed caretakers—of modern times. Health-care professionals in general have a responsibility to avoid misleading themselves or the public about what the services offer or can do.

The perspective of Police

Unlike the Medical and Nursing professions, which have given little thought to the training of doctors and nurses to face the problems of death and bereavement, the Police have seriously attempted to deal with these issues in training recruits. What follows attempts to summarise current practice.

Since Police involvement with death and bereavement is chiefly in the area of sudden, accidental and violent death, training is related to the role of policemen in such situations and their dealings with the public. This includes: experience of contact with dead bodies, giving death messages, follow-up after bereavement, dealing with requests for post mortems, giving information about death-procedure.

All cases of sudden, accidental or violent death are referred to the Traffic Enquiry Department rather than the CID. This reorganisation was undertaken because the majority of accidental deaths are from road traffic accidents, and also to avoid the embarrassment of the family which involvement of the CID sometimes caused.

Once the police have been informed of a death the doctor is called. In the case of sudden death the doctor may not have seen the patient for a while and he may hesitate to give a death certificate. Sometimes permission may have to be sought from the relatives for a post-mortem, but the tendency now is for post-mortems to be avoided if possible and a 'View and Grant' to be given instead.

In all cases of sudden or accidental death the policeman on the beat is first sent along. He has the responsibility to search the body, and to satisfy himself that there is nothing suspicious. He then accompanies the body to the mortuary, fills in the appropriate forms and completes the death register. People are sometimes found dead in the street—heart failure and strokes being the commonest causes rather than violence or accidents. When this happens the policeman may have the responsibility of informing the next-of-kin and may have to accompany them to the mortuary to identify the body.

It is the policeman's job to knock on doors and try to find out tactfully where the dead person has lived and about their family and background. It is police policy to avoid giving death messages directly to the next-of-kin and the attempt is made to enlist the help of a friend or relative to tell them. In this way the bereaved can be given immediate help and support. Where a direct police approach is necessary two officers usually go together (sometimes including a woman PC). This means that one can remain with the relative or family while the other attends to immediate practical arrangements. Police policy is against giving death messages on the telephone and whenever possible these are given face to face. In this way the circumstances of the bereaved can be observed and help obtained if necessary. If there is a police enquiry, the policeman who gives the original message is usually required to maintain contact and liaison with the family throughout the whole period of the enquiry.

Police training is consciously geared to these various tasks which policemen have in handling dead bodies and communicating with bereaved relatives. For example, because police officers have the unpleasant duty of having to search the bodies of victims of sudden death or road traffic accidents, care is taken to introduce new recruits by a visit to the police mortuary where they are encouraged to touch and handle a dead body and to talk about their reactions to this experience. Police Officers are prepared in this way to face and examine their feelings and reactions in the presence of death (and often mutilated remains). Ability to do so is seen to be important in relation to handling relatives who have to be taken to the mortuary to identify the remains. These visits are rehearsed and officers instructed in the proper procedure and appropriate behaviour. Associated with this training is a policy that young trainees should always be accompanied to the scene of a fatal accident or sudden death by a senior officer whose job it is to instruct the trainee in the appropriate action to be taken.

Special attention is given in training to the communication of death messages. In the Police Training school use is made of simulated accidents to give trainees experience of communicating bad news. The use of role-play and appropriate de-briefing afterwards is recommended. In addition trainees are expected to be accompanied by a senior officer when communicating a death message. In the first instance they observe their senior performing this duty, later their own performance is monitored by the senior officer. It was stressed that so far as possible arrangements must be made to ensure that the bereaved are not left alone after being told, and that

36

in the first instance the policeman must try to communicate the message via a close relative or friend who can remain to give support afterwards. (The care taken over communication of death messages by the police contrasted with the virtual absence of any training in these matters for doctors and nurses. While the handling of death messages by nurses and doctors, particularly hospital doctors, was severely criticised by CRUSE and the 'consumer' group of bereaved persons (see Appendix), the police were frequently commended by the same sources for their exemplary handling of these difficult situations.)

Other matters with a bearing on bereavement to which attention is given in police training are: the appropriate consideration for bereaved people in the case of a police enquiry—where it is recommended that the same officer or officers should maintain contact with the family to give support and advice; secondly, the question of requesting permission for a post-mortem—where the need for a sympathetic approach is emphasised; and finally the giving of information about legal and other procedures relating to death (e.g. in relation to death certificates, registration and claims for benefits) —where it is emphasised that it is the policeman's duty to be properly informed so that he can give reliable and accurate advice. (Once again the lack of concern for follow-up of the bereaved, insensitivity about PM requests and general ignorance of death procedure on the part of hospital staff were criticised by CRUSE and the Bereaved Group.)

The role of the Funeral Director

Funeral Directors are likewise concerned with practical matters and the alleviation of distress to the bereaved. They emphasised that funerals serve three general purposes: First, to fulfil the legal and health requirements for the proper disposal of remains. (Funeral Directors perform this service on behalf of the relatives, the local authority and the state.) Second, funerals have a function in relation to the ritualisation of grief and mourning and the alleviation of distress through the release of emotion, as well as providing a social occasion or context for the expression of public sympathy or support for the bereaved. Third, funerals are conducted in accordance with the wishes of the bereaved family or the last wishes of the deceased, providing an appropriate form or ceremony where family and mourners can 'pay their last respects' to the dead whether in religious terms or otherwise.

The Funeral Directors saw their basic function as that of alleviating distress by acting on behalf of the relatives and relieving them of making funeral arrangements in the immediate shock and aftermath of a death. Their tasks might include making enquiries on behalf of the bereaved from doctors or other officials, giving general advice and undertaking payment of immediate expenses in connection with the burial or cremation. Their function was to alleviate distress by good public relations work on behalf of the family, by acting as a buffer between the family and officialdom and by efficient execution of their wishes in relation to the deceased. They also saw themselves as having a responsibility to protect people from making rash decisions concerning the size and expense of funerals.

The main areas in which Funeral Directors considered that professional services to the dying and the bereaved could be improved, related to the following: information about death procedure, certification of deaths, post-mortems and death-grants, etc.

General ignorance of death-procedure was cited as a cause of much confusion and distress to the bereaved. Dealing with this ignorance was seen to be the responsibility of several professions— for example, lawyers in relation to wills and estates, doctors and nurses in relation to the certification and registration of deaths, social workers in relation to Insurance, Social Security, Death Grants and other benefits, the police in relation to the need for investigation of sudden, accidental or violent deaths. The fact that Funeral Directors have to advise informally on these matters was accepted as inevitable but undesirable as the misunderstanding and ignorance should be removed before people have need to consult a Funeral Director.

Doctors and particularly nursing staff are often inadequately informed about the various certificates which are required for the registration of a death, for burial or cremation. The result is that they are unable to advise people correctly what they should do once a death has been certified. It was contended that doctors seldom explain to relatives what is written on the death certificate and that this can cause serious misunderstanding and distress. 'People tend to be admitted to hospital with euphemisms and die of real diseases.' Delays in completing the necessary paper-work can cause delays and uncertainty in completing funeral arrangements. People are not informed that a death can be registered at home—in either the district where the deceased resided or died. This results in relatives sometimes having to make long and unnecessary trips to the city to do what they can do in their own town.

The issue of the insensitivity of medical staff in obtaining permission for post-mortems or removal of organs for transplant purposes was remarked upon, as well as the distress to relatives viewing remains by inconsiderate post-mortem incisions. There was considerable doubt expressed about whether all PMs were strictly necessary—particularly in the case of infants, still births and the elderly.

These areas of avoidable distress emphasised by Police and Funeral Directors were considered to be important for the study of professional attitudes and values in the care of the dying and the bereaved, first because something practical can be done about them, but second, because they illustrate areas of insensitivity in the attitudes of the caring professions to the problems of the dying and the bereaved. (For further detailed comment and recommendations see Appendix.)

The perspective of CRUSE and the bereaved

Critical feedback on Professional services from the Bereaved. The group of widows, widowers and bereaved parents which was specially convened for this purpose prepared a detailed set of recommendations for the improvement of terminal care and support for the bereaved.

In relation to Hospital Doctors, criticisms focused on inadequate communication with the dying and with relatives. There is a need for doctors to tell the truth and not side-step issues. The communication of diagnoses and prognoses was handled in a patronising and condescending manner. While in some circumstances the doctor was justified in not telling the patient that he was dying, in general patients 'know the score' and are not helped by deception or equivocation. The communication with relatives following a death was poorly handled in most cases.

In relation to General Practitioners the chief complaints were lack of consideration in moving elderly sick patients from home to hospital, or from one hospital to another, and the fact that few GPs visit their patients in hospital when they are dying. The issue of communication was of central importance—both in communication around the dying patient and in maintaining contact following bereavement.

Nurses were described as too eager to take over all the nursing functions, leaving the relatives with little to do, feeling excluded and useless. It was important in relation to subsequent bereavement that close relatives or significant others should be allowed, where possible, to minister to the needs of their loved ones. The lack of understanding of the need for privacy in hospital when someone is dying was a matter of concern to bereaved relatives. Nurses too were criticised for the delivery of death-messages—especially the telephone call simply saying So-and-so had died, without establishing whether the recipient of the information was alone, had the

39

means to get to the hospital, etc. In the hospital, all too often nurses give the bereaved relatives a cup of tea and then send them on their way without enquiring whether they have someone to drive them home or have anyone to go to.

Social Workers have perhaps little part to play at the moment of death, but they could be of great assistance in helping relatives when they are told bad news—either when coping with the shock of a fatal diagnosis, or in coping with immediate grief-reactions. Similarly Social Workers could be more active in the follow-up of bereaved people—particularly where the bereavement is protracted or where the death causes serious complications in the life of the family.

In relation to the Clergy their ministry to the dying and the bereaved can be of great value, not in an officious clerical role, but being an independent professional willing to listen and give practical advice and assistance. For some people the spiritual ministry of a clergyman might be important, but the majority of people turn to the clergyman because of his assumed familiarity with death and, in the case of bereavement, his knowledge of how things might be done decently and in good order.

These criticisms and reactions of the bereaved are mentioned because they represent another angle from which the phenomenon of bereavement needs to be examined and defined. No particular claims are made for the validity of the views expressed by this limited sample of bereaved persons, but whether universally valid or not, they represent significant reactions to death and bereavement—views which need to be taken into account in attempting to achieve an over-view of professional/patient reactions in the context of death and bereavement.

Dealing with the emotional and practical problems of bereavement. Two different kinds of problems require different kinds of management: (i) the problems of bereavement and its psychological consequences, and (ii) the practical problems created by the loss of a spouse or close companion.

CRUSE has evolved its own ways of giving both kinds of assistance. As a self-help organisation for widows, CRUSE seeks to help widows find their way back to a purposeful life and back into the community in whatever way is appropriate and helpful to each family's circumstances.

In discussing a wide variety of cases with CRUSE members a number of general observations were made, which we summarise here because they serve both to illustrate the nature of bereavement and the problems faced by professionals and lay-organisations in helping the bereaved.

Presenting problems. CRUSE members identified these as follows: most come seeking company and relief from loneliness; many come with practical problems, including health problems; a smaller number come for counselling and an opportunity to talk confidentially about their loss or their emotional problems in getting over it.

Referrals. Most who approach CRUSE are self-referrals. Sometimes widows are referred by Social Workers, GPs or other agencies. Many are referred by other widows or recently bereaved friends. A small number come because they have read the publicity. The majority come for the social activities and tend to be widows of long standing.

Communicating with the recently bereaved. This was generally recognised to be very difficult. Recently bereaved widows show a massive defensiveness against the possibility of being hurt again, and tend to withdraw into themselves for a while. They may later begin to feel the burden of their isolation and seek company. This withdrawal may have alienated old friends, and, in any case widows often seek new friends because old friendships may have too many painful associations. These facts make it difficult to communicate relevant information about available support and services to the recently bereaved. Their initial state of shock, confusion and grief makes it difficult for them to remember information given to them by their GP or minister, or undertaker. (It was felt that advice about organisations such as CRUSE and other forms of available professional help should be given at a later stage in bereavement.)

Normal and abnormal grief. CRUSE members were unanimous that people need time to grieve. As one case worker expressed it: 'They need a quiet time (knowing that support is there and available if needed), time to weep over their letters and photographs, time to explore their grief and work it out. Above all they need to be free of the intrusive people, professional or lay, who are over-anxious to help and interfere. Weeping is a very healing thing. People should be allowed to weep, should be encouraged to weep and left alone too sometimes, to weep on their own. Scots mothers are taught not to weep in public—like Spartan mothers—but it gnaws at their vitals.'

The case workers observed that there seems to be a relation between inability to weep and the almost compulsive need to talk, and said that they often remarked that a widow was getting better, getting over her bereavement, if she was not talking so much. The need to talk out their grief rather than cry it out often means that such widows make unreasonable demands on individual caring

41

persons who try to help them. The inability to weep also seems to express itself in extreme restlessness—which can drive friends and helpers to distraction. They seem to find it necessary to be always active, as if they were unconsciously looking for something lost. This, some of the widows observed, seemed worst when a woman had nursed her husband for a long time and has perhaps done a lot of her grieving before his death, and then finds herself with nothing to do, with no focus for her activity and unable to grieve openly any more. Such women feel guilty for not grieving more, and worry that they perhaps failed to do enough for their husbands. It was stressed that the form taken by the grief reaction often has a lot to do with the nature of the past relationship—where the relationship had been a happy and fulfilled one bereavement was got over quickly, where the relationship was unhappy or where the widow had been very dependent on her husband the grief-reaction could be prolonged and complicated. Anniversaries were mentioned as presenting people with particular emotional problems. These seasonal reminders could trigger off renewed grief or depression and it was stressed that people need particular emotional support at such times. CRUSE members try to make special efforts to include in their social activities members approaching anniversaries and festive occasions.

Two kinds of abnormal grief-reactions were mentioned: first the obvious cases where bereavement precipitates major mental breakdown, or a sufficient degree of mental disturbance to warrant psychiatric intervention, and second, the problems of the dependent individual who seems chronically unable to cope with the experience of loss. In the first type of case CRUSE members had no hesitation in referring the individual to a psychiatrist. In the second type of case they were less certain. Such individuals were often referred back to them for help. Some they felt were partly suffering from iatrogenic complications of bereavement: 'Doctors have a lot to answer for, for so readily prescribing pills for stress.'

Practical problems and consequences of bereavement. CRUSE members stressed that the loss of a wife or husband was often a kind of multiple bereavement. A woman may lose her husband— who also handled the finances, helped to discipline the children, was a good handy-man, handled matters relating to their house and property etc. The more dependent a wife is on her husband or vice versa, the more acute will be the practical problems she faces when confronted by the loss of someone on whom she has relied for help with day-to-day problems. In particular widows and widowers find difficulty coping alone with children and find it difficult to socialise without an accepted escort. Dealing with financial and legal matters is a cause of difficulty to many widows, housekeeping and domestic chores to widowers.

Bereavement often means loss of economic status, with the loss of the husband's earnings and associated status. The relative poverty in which widows may find themselves—even if only temporarily while the estate is being wound up—can cause great distress and embarrassment.

Bereavement frequently means giving up the family home and moving to a new and unfamiliar social environment—with its associated problems and difficulties in achieving integration in the new community. This tends not only to isolate the widow more but means that she has to initiate all the new contacts in her new environment. In a minority of cases moving may be beneficial not only making practical arrangements easier if the house is smaller, nearer to relatives, in a more convenient neighbourhood etc., but it may also encourage the widow to make a new life for herself and begin again.

In general the overwhelming practical problem of the bereaved was felt to be loneliness and learning to cope alone after many years of close companionship and sharing of responsibility. 'How to cope with loneliness and how to begin again on your own — those are the problems. You don't want to have to go out and do things on your own, yet you don't want to be pitied. It is an impossible dilemma. If you seek for companionship you seem to be asking to be pitied, yet you cannot overcome loneliness on your own.'

Discussion and identification of problems

Arising out of the Working Group's discussions with the Police, Funeral Directors, CRUSE and the specially convened group of Bereaved persons, it was generally agreed that the preparation of health-care professionals to deal with death is unsatisfactory, and that criticism of their ignorance of death procedure is probably justified. Training of health-care professionals to care for the dying and the bereaved is inadequate, and the Working Group decided to set up special sub-committees representing the Medical, Nursing, Social Work professions and Ministers of Religion to investigate this question and to make recommendations for the improvement of professional training. The reports of these sub-committees are contained in Appendix 1, and further recommendations from Funeral Directors, CRUSE and the Bereaved Group are contained in the Appendix.

The most important problems with moral implications which were identified in discussion are the following: i) the question of whether it is desirable for bereavement to be treated as an illness; ii) the problems and stresses faced by the professional confronted by the over-demanding, chronically bereaved patient; iii) the danger of medicalising bereavement, with the consequent iatrogenic complications of dependency and excessive drug use; iv) the questions raised by bereavement management of where to draw the limits to professional responsibility.

i) There was considerable disagreement about the treatment of bereavement as an illness. The bereaved, who usually need help some time after the initial crisis of grief is past, often find it difficult to approach the doctor for help unless they present with some illness. The bereaved also frequently find it reassuring to be told that bereavement is like an illness, which follows a definite course, has a finite duration and is something from which you eventually recover. Further the fact that bereavement is so often associated with deterioration of health means that it is helpful for the doctor to be encouraged to see the bereaved person as a potential patient in need of help, and for the bereaved individual to see his physical and psychological symptoms as part of the normal course of bereavement, or his more abnormal psychological reactions as treatable medical complaints.

On the negative side it was suggested that rather than specifically medical attention the kind of help needed by the bereaved, to cope with loneliness, guilt and depression, is usually someone to talk to. The danger is that because the doctor is probably the most readily available professional in the community, and because bereavement symptoms mimic illness-patterns, the bereaved person will be encouraged to adopt the patient-role and accept the illness-label in order to 'earn' attention and the suspension of responsibilities, the privileges of care and moratorium for recovery associated with being ill. Likewise the risk is that the busy doctor will have recourse to the prescription pad, treat the presenting symptoms, or refer the person on to a Social Worker, Minister or Psychiatrist, rather than make time to discuss the person's bereavement with them. Being 'ill' legitimises the bereaved in seeking medical and professional help, but it also creates the risks associated with the medicalisation of bereavement, the pressure on people to become patient-dependants at a time when they are dependency-prone.

ii) The problems faced by professionals in dealing with over-demanding clients are most commonly associated with individuals suffering from some kind of bereavement. There was general endorsement of the Social Worker's view that most professionals find it difficult to cope with such individuals and find it even more difficult to admit when they are not coping and need the help of others. The tendency to 'pass the buck' and refer the patient on was observed to be a common strategy for dealing with 'problem patients / clients', rather than frank consultation with colleagues. It was remarked that Social Workers are beginning to learn to ask for help and to provide support for one another. Doctors, nurses and ministers were thought to be inclined to try to cope on their own and to be less good at providing support for one another. As one doctor remarked: 'We haven't built in to our caring community a way of admitting our own inadequacy in the face of death and bereavement.'

iii) The tendency towards the medicalisation of bereavement, with the attendant doctor-dependency and excessive drug use which this creates, was a problem of professional attitudes as much as a matter of public expectations. It is not only doctors who are inappropriately or inadequately trained to help the bereaved, but as people increasingly turn to other professionals for help with their bereavement problems so they too are often responsible for creating dependency in such individuals through inappropriate management. The temptation to say that bereavement is not a responsibility of professionals but should be the responsibility of lay organisations or the community was real, but not a satisfactory solution. With increasing urbanisation of society such problems are likely to be relegated to professionals—even if only in organising and co-ordinating appropriate support. The central problem was that professionals should be taught to understand the nature of bereavement both in its normal and abnormal forms and should be given a better understanding of the complex practical problems faced by bereaved individuals. In this way doctors, nurses, social workers, ministers and other caring individuals would be helped to recognise where it is appropriate for them to intervene and / or devise appropriate responses to both the emotional and practical needs of those who seek their assistance.

iv) The fact that bereavement is a process which may take a long time, that the bereaved tend to make considerable demands on the time and resources of professionals when they become involved in care, and the fact that the problems of the bereaved may be intractable, all raise problems for the concerned professional about the scope and limits of his professional responsibilities. Dilemmas about the limits of care were considered to be particularly difficult to resolve, especially for the idealistic and conscientious individual, as they involve conflicts between immediate practical responsibilities and more general religious and moral responsibilities. The

E　　　　　　　45

individual caring person is left uncertain as to how much responsibility he must accept for the bereaved, how much of the responsibility should be passed back to the community, and how much the bereaved should be encouraged to accept responsibility for themselves.

SUGGESTED READING FOR CHAPTER THREE
The studies listed in the Bibliography under Carlson (1970), Cartwright (1973), Edinburgh Consumer Group (1976), Elfert (1975), Freud (1917), Gibson (1974), Gorer (1965), Kübler-Ross (1970 and 1975), Kutscher (1969), Leared (1974), Maddison & Raphael, Marks (1976), Parkes (1964 and 1972), Pearson (1969), Pincus (1976), Rees, Schmale, Stephen (1972), Torrie (1970.)

PART TWO

Case Studies in Moral Dilemmas

FOUR

The Ethics of Intervention in Terminal Care

IN CHAPTER ONE four kinds of moral dilemmas relating to professional involvement in the pre-death phase were identified. In this chapter these dilemmas are further examined and discussed against the background of a specific case. The case is an example of a single profession involvement and a simple 'contract' in which only the patient suffering from inoperable cancer and his GP were involved. The fact that the patient's wife was not consulted, that a conservative form of management was adopted, and that the GP chose a course of minimal interference in the patient's life, provoked much controversy.

In the course of discussion the Working Group distinguished between a 'minimalist' and 'maximalist' approach to terminal care observing the advantages and limitations of both these views of professional responsibility to the dying. Further, different models for the doctor/patient or professional/client relationship were considered, namely: the traditional approach based on *Professional Code*, the increasingly popular *Contract* model, and the conception of an inter-personal *Covenant*. The relevance of each to relationships with the dying, was discussed. It was recognised that the professional's view of his function, e.g. to cure or care, and his view of his professional duties would vary according to whether he adopted a 'minimalist' or 'maximalist' approach to intervention in terminal care, and according to how he conceived his 'contract' with the dying patient/client/person.

What is meant by 'the ethics of intervention'

Ethics is the study of the moral pre-suppositions which govern our actions and guide our decisions in daily life. There are two kinds of circumstances which may cause us to reflect critically upon our moral presuppositions, namely when some other person challenges our accepted moral beliefs, or when we face a crisis of some kind.

When this occurs we may respond by simply and dogmatically reaffirming them, or we may subject our moral beliefs to criticism and may modify or reject them. More commonly, however, we are driven to seek some rational justification for them, we attempt to clarify the grounds on which we normally base our moral decisions —decisions which we might otherwise take fairly automatically. Similarly, when we face a crisis, in which we have to decide between difficult alternatives, we are usually compelled to re-examine the presuppositions on which we ordinarily act. While in the philosophical study of ethics we seek deliberately, calmly and systematically to study our moral presuppositions and the kinds of rational justification which can be offered for them, in everyday life we may be driven by personal challenge or crisis to attempt the same sort of thing.

The discovery that a patient/client/friend is dying is typically the kind of situation which prompts a re-examination of the moral presuppositions governing personal and professional relationships, because it represents both a crisis in such relationships and because the death itself is a personal challenge to our moral beliefs.

The identification of Pre-Death is important, as we have seen, not only for scientific reasons, or in the interests of accurate description, but more basically because of the practical and moral decisions which flow from it. The death of a patient has an effect on the morale of health-care professionals, because morale is founded upon the moral values and beliefs which provide the pre-suppositions for action, and these may be called in question by a death. The death may raise doubts about the kind of care and management the person has been given, but also more disquieting doubts for the individual about the value of what he is doing. If these are not discussed and examined they remain to haunt and disturb the minds of those who have the responsibility of caring for the dying, providing undercurrents of tension and anxiety in dealings with patients and in inter-professional relationships. The justification for examining some of these questions is not their academic interest or importance, but rather that the open discussion of the moral doubts, anxieties and dilemmas associated with terminal care can have beneficial effects for professional morale and patient care.

The moral dilemmas associated with medical and other-professional intervention in terminal care are the subject of this discussion of 'the ethics of intervention'. What is the proper role of the doctor/nurse/social worker/minister in caring for the dying? What freedom ought the patient to have in deciding the form of terminal care provided? To what extent must confidentiality be strictly maintained? Has the patient a right to know his condition? Is the professional bound to accept the increased responsibilities imposed on him by the requirements of terminal care? How far must the professional take responsibility for the patient without consulting or without being able to consult him, and how far has he a responsibility to help the patient to face the reality of his impending death? How far should the individual become personally involved with the dying patient and how far should he be willing to take independent decisions e.g. about telling the patient the truth, or in terminating investigations and treatment?

Not all these questions are discussed in the present chapter, and for that reason 'the ethics of intervention' could be taken as a title for the whole investigation of professional responsibilities in caring for the dying and the bereaved. Different views on the appropriate nature and extent of professional intervention in terminal care and the question of the most appropriate way of conceiving the 'contract' with the dying patient are two issues which are discussed in some detail. The other questions are touched upon, but also recur as themes in later discussions.

Case presentation

The following case was intended to open up discussion of the above-mentioned areas of moral conflict in terminal care, and to illustrate how some of the issues arise directly and others only indirectly in practice. The case was presented by a *general practitioner*.

'Mr Macintosh'

'Mr Macintosh' A 60 year old taxi-driver, with a wife and one married son. (His wife a patient of another doctor in a different practice.)

Mid-December: Came in for investigation because of cough and spitting small amounts of blood. Signs of acute chest infection. Smokes 15 a day.

Late December: Still coughing blood in small amounts. Normal chest X-ray. Suspicion of lung cancer.

Early January: Symptoms persist. Refer to chest physician. Confirmed diagnosis.

Early February: Diagnosis of inoperable cancer. Patient waiting to go to hospital for radio-therapy.
'I'm in a very bad way, my chest's in a mess.'
'Is it hopeless, Doctor?'
Explored this a little. 'What do you mean by hopeless?'

Early March: Very weak after radio-therapy.

Late March: Depressed but not suicidal. (Difficult stage in treatment.) Natural physiological or pathological process?

Late April: Didn't go on holiday. Nocturnal cough. More

coughing up of blood in small amounts. Needing explanation of worsening symptoms. Explained as reaction to therapy. Given remedy for cough.

Early July: Still coughing but not too bad. Plans to go on post-poned holiday.

Late July: Returned home from holiday on Saturday. Seen by partner. Admitted to hospital the next day. Dies four days later (without my knowledge).

Comment by G P. This was a case of a simple GP/Patient contract—a single profession involvement. It raises questions about whether the GP's contract is with the individual patient or with the patient and his family. Should I have involved the wife who was someone else's patient? The official contract of the GP is to provide general medical care, not to get involved with third parties. This obviously can lead to difficulties.

You may be critical of my management of this case, but I felt that he had failed me. I thought I was doing well on continuity and then he went and got worse when I wasn't around. There are difficulties in maintaining continuity of care in the modern group practice.

Comment by Social Worker: 'How little is known about the family and the patient's life-situation. We need to ask how much information is required to provide a productive service. The definition of the scope of the 'problem' is relative to the kind of knowledge available. In the case of Mr Macintosh who had the problem? He had the cancer? Maybe his wife had the problem!'

Respect for the rights of others requires that we know their needs. The patient and his wife are functionally inseparable. The wife had rights. Was it convenient for the GP to restrict the scope of his responsibility by ignoring them? One wants to ask whether inter-GP confidentiality provides an excuse for stalling. Who else can initiate an approach to the wife, but the GP? There are bound to be many practical problems—rights to benefits etc. The wife was entitled to be informed.

Knowledge and expertise entail responsibilities for the professional who has them. These relate to the rights of patients/clients to adequate information so that they in turn can take responsible decisions. What needs were expressed or clues given by the patient that were ignored? Whose responsibility was it to share the prognosis with this man? The GP? The Hospital? There was displacement of responsibility between GP and hospital. The case illustrates how the definition of the patient's 'problem' and the 'management' of 'the patient' is regulated by the control of available information—either by limiting the amount of information sought or controlling the amount of information given.

Illustrative Discussion

There was polarization in the discussion between the doctors on the one hand and social workers and district nurses on the other. The GP took the view that intervention must be asked for and that the patient's rights take precedence over those of other family members. The social workers and district nurses took the view that the family unit is important and that they have a right to be involved in decisions relating to terminal care and ought to be offered the help and support of other services.

Intervention or Interference. It emerged in discussion that people's 'problems' tend to be conceived and defined by professionals, and presented for solution within what the professional considers to be his area of competence. Doctors were accused of so restricting the definition of their area of clinical responsibility that they often tend to ignore important social and psychological dimensions of a case. Social workers were accused by doctors of taking as their diocese an area which embraces the whole life of the patient/client, including the people around them, and this it was contended could lead to unnecessary interference in the lives of people. However, all agreed that 'problems' must be defined sufficiently specifically to be capable of some kind of solution, and that professionals should not go about attempting to solve insoluble problems.

Psychiatrist: Is the GP's contract with the patient or with the patient and his family? Social workers would appear to say 'the whole family'. How much have we a right to know about a patient? It could be argued that the more we know the more we understand. However, if there was intervention between the GP and the wife's doctor, then great care would be needed. It might be construed as interference by the family or 'poaching' by the other doctor.

Nurse. Why then do we talk of the 'Family Unit' if intervention with the family is unacceptable? There must be inter-liaison between doctor and parents in the treatment of a child. Why not in the treatment of terminally ill patients?

Psychiatrist. In dealing with his depression it might have been helpful to consult the wife and other family members.

Lawyer. The question is whether he came to the doctor for help with a specific problem or whether he is asking 'for the whole works'?

52

Physician. The question is whether he needs 'the whole works'.

Social Worker. How do you know unless you investigate? Must everything depend on the sensitivity or insensitivity of the GP?

GP. While the patient is ambulant and seeing the GP I feel that the doctor must leave the initiative to the patient and not be too interventionist with the family.

District Nurse. The man in the surgery is in an artificial situation. If he was seen by the doctor at home or in hospital it is likely that the wife would have been involved and the question of who was who's patient would be unimportant. The doctor knows he is going to die. Supportive intervention is needed if proper terminal care is to be arranged.

Lawyer. But what right do you have to pester the wife and family, unless asked for help?

Chaplain. The sad thing is that when intervention would have been unquestioningly justified, the doctor was not there . . . a damn sad ending.

During the course of further discussion the different attitudes to intervention illustrated here were characterised as '*minimalist*' and '*maximalist*'. The cautious attitude of the GP and the Lawyer were described as minimalist, because they were responsive to expressed need and did not seek out undeclared dependency. The 'maximalist' approach was identified with the attitudes of the District Nurse, Social Worker and Psychiatrist. Their approach was seen to be based on a comprehensive view of the ideal form of terminal care—in which patient and family co-operate with a variety of professionals in the health-care team to provide the best service to the dying patient. Protagonists of the 'minimalist' approach alleged that there are risks involved in the 'maximalist' approach—that it is too intrusive and that the rights of patients and family members are compromised in the interests of 'total care'. They also maintained that a 'minimalist' approach to intervention avoids the danger of over-medicalising terminal care and leaves people less dependent on the health-care professionals. Conversely, it was maintained that the 'maximalist' view encourages full consultation between different professionals and between individual professionals and the family unit, including the patient, whereas it was maintained that the 'minimalist' view encourages the individual professionals, particularly doctors, to retain exclusive control of their patients.

The single-profession, one-contract case is closer to the norm than the ideal of total care offered by the Primary Medical Care Team. 'The minimalist approach is appropriate to what actually happened, the maximalist view to what perhaps ought to happen.

We have to distinguish between the awkward facts of the real world and the hoped-for ideal of total care.' If the professional is encouraged to expand out of this minimalist definition of his role and duties, in response to specific needs or crises, e.g. in undertaking additional responsibilities relative to dying patients, then he tends to feel insecure and may retreat back into the minimalist interpretation of his responsibilities if faced with unreasonable demands from patients, or threatened conflict with other professionals. The penumbra of vagueness which tends to develop around professional roles in the situation of expanded responsibility in a team approach to terminal care, may be an advantage in breaking down professional barriers, but it may also become an area of uncertainty and moral conflict for individuals and between different professionals who become confused about their roles.

The actions of the doctor are predicated upon the one-to-one nature of his relationship with his patient. This tends to deter complicating extensions out of this one-to-one relationship. The social worker is willing to initiate investigations to enable clients to recruit help as required, because it is part of the social worker's function to co-ordinate help and resources for those in need. However the social worker may impute problems and over-zealously seek out undeclared needs. Ministers may confine their attention to the spiritual needs of the individual alone, but are more likely to become involved with family and relatives for religious and moral reasons. They are likely to endorse a maximalist approach to terminal care and for the same reason may risk becoming spiritual 'do-gooders'.

While the choice between 'minimalist' and 'maximalist' attitudes to intervention in terminal care was seen to be important in principle, it was emphasised that in practice the pattern of care is dictated more by the nature of the place where the patient is treated and the resources available, e.g. in the home, in hospital or in a hospice. Morals may be more affected by institutions than by professional attitudes and values, although the reform of the former may depend on the latter. In practice the availability of a social worker or the question of whether the wife is involved in decisions about terminal care may depend on the context where the patient is treated. Similarly the transition from 'pre-death' to 'dying' may involve different sets of morals coming into operation, the point at which this takes place being determined on technical grounds by the doctor.

Confidentiality. The problems of the doctor/patient and inter-professional confidentiality raised by this case were discussed briefly. The traditional confidential relationship between doctor and patient may change subtly when the patient is dying. This may affect the way the doctor views his responsibilities to his patient, in relation to the communication of prognosis and in obtaining informed consent for continuing or discontinuing investigations and treatment. He may feel inhibited from discussing the implications of a bad prognosis with the patient because he wishes to help the patient sustain a hopeful attitude, or because he is unwilling to face the emotional complications to his relationship with the patient which may result from telling him the truth. He may feel it is unfair to confront the patient with choices about his treatment and may feel obliged to accept personal responsibility for such decisions. Alternatively he may be afraid that the patient may make unacceptable demands if allowed the opportunity to decide what should be done.

Forms of terminal care which involve a hospital-based or community-based inter-professional health-care team, presuppose a wide interpretation of the duty to maintain confidentiality. The extended confidentiality which includes the sharing of vital information with other members of the team 'in the best interests of the patient', is justified on the grounds that the patient is dying and that the extra-ordinary situation makes it legitimate to compromise the demands of strict confidentiality. Whether this is ever morally justified without the patient's consent was questioned, but it was admitted that in practice extended confidentiality is less the exception than the rule.

Chairman. Are the moral grounds for not having involved the family that the doctor/patient contract is personal and confidential and to have involved them would have infringed the patient's rights. Is that right?

GP. Essentially.

Social Worker. I would see the wife as having rights here too.

Lawyer. But she failed to exercise them. It was up to her.

GP. To have involved the wife and family would have meant asking the patient. While he accepted the diagnosis as fatal he still had his hope of going camping in Wester Ross. I didn't want to shatter his dream of doing this. Confidentiality as between doctor and husband and wife is a difficult one.

Social Worker. Clearly you could not involve her until you had spoken to him. You had to first have an honest and open discussion with him. Was that not really necessary in the interests of good terminal care?

GP. The truth was not evaded, but trying to find out his perception of the situation seemed important. He hoped for a lengthy remission. There is danger in being too extreme . . . the truth is important, but pragmatic leeway is needed in deciding whether the patient should be confronted with the whole truth.

Chairman. Is it a technical decision when it is appropriate to tell the truth? What is the basis of this . . . practical necessity or what? Is there not an underlying obligation to tell the truth?

Chaplain. He was an hospital in-patient for a while. What if the wife had phoned up then and asked for information?

GP. I would take a hard line on confidentiality. I would have said that the husband would need to be involved in any decision. Doctors can appear to override the rule of confidentiality but I think it's a bedrock principle and almost an absolute.

Chaplain. You acted unilaterally here. The human problems in such cases affect other people and other professionals on the team. Where do you think they come in and what about confidentiality?

GP. If the timing is usual (this chap let me down) . . . then it is the practical purposes of intervention of others that counts. If I had known of his Church contacts I might have talked to the minister when he seemed to be at the stage of needing help. The problems would have been discussed with the team (Social Worker, District Nurse, etc.) when practical care was needed.

Chaplain. When the true nature of the patient's condition is concealed then it is difficult for the minister, for example, to become involved. What inhibits you from coming clean?

GP. Here I didn't clearly know . . . that is the point. Prognosis in terms of time is difficult until it is obvious. Confidentiality within the medical team is easy but with others, e.g. ministers . . . can be more difficult. I believe in openness (this is my personal philosophy) but in an optimistic form. The time to come clean is when it is obvious. There is a need to reassure that you are going to be there, available. To tell too early may make it too difficult, e.g. here the caravan trip.

Chairman. Your view arises from construing the doctor/ patient relationship simply as a one-to-one relationship. You doctors seem to agree on practicality and pragmatism. That means you are in control.

The chief point to emerge from discussion was the relativity of the concept of confidentiality in different social contexts. Social changes, for example, changes in the status of women and a tendency towards patient-initiated intervention require a more flexible approach to confidentiality. Changes in the organisation of health-care services also mean that the traditional conception of confidentiality, based as it is on an intimate personal relationship with a particular doctor, needs to be re-examined in the light of new developments such as Group Practices, Deputising Services and the tendency for greater involvement of inter-disciplinary teams, particularly in the context of terminal care

The traditional values of privacy, trust and secrecy on which the rule of confidentiality is based remain important both on moral and practical grounds. On moral grounds they serve as the means to protect the rights of the patient in his situation of exposed vulnerability and need, and they also provide the basis for the doctor's moral authority. On practical grounds the efficacy of 'the drug: doctor' (Balint, M., 1957), depends in a fundamental way on the maintenance of a meaningful confidential relationship with the patient. The confidence and truthfulness, which are possible only in a confidential relationship, are essential to both the moral and therapeutic character of the doctor/patient relation.

The question of the confidentiality of medical records has become a problem as an increasing number of people have access to confidential material, as data storage and retrieval becomes mechanised and as a situation of extended confidentiality increasingly obtains for reasons of necessity in multi-professional health-care. It becomes increasingly urgent for institutional safeguards for patients' rights to be developed, and for people to be better informed about what use is likely to be made of their medical records. There is a need for the limits of confidentiality to be more explicitly defined with each patient, and their consent obtained for the communication of confidential information.

The nature of the doctor/patient contract

Chairman. We seem to have fallen in with current fashion of using the word 'contract' for the relationship between doctor and patient. Social workers use the term a lot, but is it really appropriate for the relationship of doctor and patient or the relationship between a chaplain and his parishioner?

Social Worker. We use the term to get away from more patronising views of professional/client relationships. A contract implies something which is formally negotiated between two independent people, as in the case of a marriage contract or a business contract, and it emphasises the dignity of the client as a user or consumer of services rather than as a dependent.

GP. That is just Social Work rhetoric. Most people who come for help are in great need and are very vulnerable. Of course it is right that their dignity should be respected, but they often are helpless dependents.

Physician. Traditionally the doctor's relationship with patients has been governed by his professional code. This is a kind of first-aid approach to the protection of patients' interests. The code guides the doctor as to what his moral and professional responsibilities are, and this is particularly important in an emergency situation or when the patient is unconscious or insane. When the doctor has to act on his own initiative and take full responsibility all he can fall back on are the codes and declarations of his profession. There can be no 'contract' in such circumstances, except in terms of implied responsibilities.

Chaplain. But that is a rather one-sided view of doctor/patient relationships, and hardly useful for the more common situation in the consulting room. Code and Contract are both equally unsatisfactory for the kind of intimate inter-personal relationship which may develop between professional and patient/client, especially in the home or terminal care ward.

2nd *GP.* I find the term 'contract' most appropriate to the consulting room. The patient comes and asks for treatment, the doctor responds to his expressed need. He does not seek out undisclosed problems. As Balint says, through a series of offers and responses on both sides a relationship is established and a form of management of the patient's complaint agreed upon. However the 'contract' is not a written contract and often should be more explicit.

Nurse. What the Chaplain says is right. The relationship you develop with a patient may be very close. 'Contract' sounds too formal. You willingly go the extra mile with some patients and with the dying are prepared to make special sacrifices. But what do you call this?

Chaplain. I was thinking that the Biblical term 'covenant' is not a bad one for the kind of personal moral commitment which is involved.

GP. Ministers may get very close to some people, but doctors do not have time or opportunity to get to know people all that well. Their knowledge is functional rather than personal and the relationship is, and perhaps ought to be, more formal.

Chaplain. I don't want to sound precious about this, but I know many doctors and nurses who are prepared to go to extraordinary lengths to help the dying—far and beyond the call of duty.

Chairman. Clearly there are different kinds of relationships possible and these may vary with different doctors and different patients, and they may vary from one context to another. The etiquette governing relationships in the home may differ from

Accident and Emergency departments in hospital, or between the consulting room and the bedside of the dying patient.

The term 'Contract' is most useful in the situation where the patient is ambulant and lucid and can approach the doctor independently to instruct medical attention. Contracts are often more imaginary than real, for they are seldom explicitly negotiated and agreed in medicine. The agreements tend to be tacit and much can be presumed upon them and both parties may feel unduly bound because so much remains implicit. Codes of practice in governing professional conduct and indirectly protecting patients' rights could not alone describe the confidential relationship of doctor and patient. The ideal of a Covenant was an attractive alternative to the more formal one-to-one contract, as it could be taken to explain the deeper sense of moral responsibility felt by professionals in certain circumstances and could also justify an approach which included other family members. There is nothing in the concept of 'Covenant' except perhaps the sense of transcendent responsibility which cannot be covered by an expanded notion of contract—where the contract is not necessarily restricted in its scope to the one-to-one professional/client relationship, where it is explicitly negotiated and is open to re-negotiation in the light of changing circumstances and needs.

Analysis of Conclusions

The ethics of different situations are different. Relief was expressed at the realisation that it was inappropriate to be looking for universal prescriptions applicable to all situations. It is far more important to explore the ethical demands of particular situations and to work out in the concrete what moral obligations are imposed on the parties involved, what opportunities exist for the expression of individual rights and to what limitations they must be subject. Thus it was emphasised that the ethical demands and opportunities vary from the consulting room to the home and from the home to the hospital.

The patient in hospital is deprived of many things which relate to his personal identity and dignity and the institutional situation subtly changes the nature and basis of confidential relationships— making the patient more dependent and depriving him of privacy. The relationships of professionals to one another is affected in various ways by decisions such as 'to settle for comfort' and whether the patient is told and allowed to share in decisions relating to his management at home or in hospital, and whether there is a sharing or non-communication about goals in management at this stage. For example, terminal care in the home or hospice tends to be more open and co-operation between doctor, district nurse, minister and others can be easier and more natural because in the nature of the case the reality is more difficult to hide. In hospital whether the patient is told or not profoundly affects the way the nursing staff relate to the patient and may make all the difference to whether the minister can make a meaningful contribution to patient support or not. Death in the home is essentially a social event, however unfortunate. Death in a hospital is essentially institutional and isolated. In the home all involved can concentrate on the needs of the dying person. In hospital there may be more than one patient dying and others in need so that the attentions of staff are divided.

In relation to the grounds and motives for intervention there appear to be two kinds of issues to be considered: general ideals; and decisions in specific situations. First there has to be a debate involving the caring professions and the public about the ideal form of terminal care—for provisions will not be made nor the appropriate institutions created unless explicit policies are formulated and official decisions taken and implemented. If it is felt to be desirable that people should be enabled to die at home, then domiciliary services need to be expanded and Primary Medical Care Teams need to be trained for effective co-operation in the provision of terminal care (Raven, R.W., 1975). If hospices for the dying are necessary with the changing pattern of mortality and increasing number of elderly in the community who are without support, then provision has to be made for the creation of such establishments and thought has to be given to the purposes and goals which they serve (Saunders, C., 1976). If the pattern of an increasing proportion of hospital deaths is to continue, then decisions have to be taken about the provision of adequate training for hospital-based medical and nursing staff in terminal care and the creation of mechanisms for more effective inter-professional co-operation (Hinton, J., 1967) and (Cartwright, A., et al, 1973).

These questions of ideal and policy are not only important for practical reasons and affect what is possible or available in a particular situation, but decisions by professionals on where they stand on these issues will affect their attitudes and expectations when they enter into a particular situation of terminal care.

That a patient has entered the 'pre-death' phase needs to be made explicit and shared with all involved (including in some instances the patient himself), the grounds for this decision need to be clearly understood and the roles of professionals and family clarified. Discussion of motives for intervention and intentions for management need to be discussed as fully as possible to ensure optimum co-operation and to avoid misunderstanding. The sharing of information with the patient and relatives, while regulated by considerations of prudence, needs to be adequate to enable them to make responsible decisions and to clarify the nature and limits of the contractual relationship and the mutual obligations involved.

Eliot Friedson, in discussing 'the social construction of illness' distinguishes between the professional construction, the lay construction, and the social organisation of illness. He points out that there may be considerable discrepancy between the conceptions and expectations of the 'sick role' of doctor, patient and society; and further that doctors, social workers and ministers may have different views of the significance of the 'illness' of the patient (Friedson, E., 1975) If this is true of illness then there is even more room for divergence of interpretation when it comes to conceptions of the nature and significance of the 'dying role'. The relevance of such sociological considerations to terminal care is not academic, although the critique of institutions and values which shape present practices may be. Professionals should be more aware of the relativity and limitations of their own institutional values, that they should become more willing to co-operate with others in the reform of existing institutions in the interests of better patient-care. Clarification of these issues clarifies too the areas in which it is appropriate for different professionals to accept responsibility for taking decisions, and where it is appropriate to take joint decisions, or to defer to the authority and expertise of another professional. The 'social construction of terminal care' need not be a mere exercise in descriptive sociology, it can become a programme, a project for the future—the goal of provision of good terminal care.

The minimalist approach. The characteristic one-to-one relationship between doctor and patient tends to be entered into cautiously and is likely to be restricted initially to the management of the patient's medical needs. Gradually as trust and confidence develop the patient may share with the doctor some of his more personal and social problems and the doctor may respond by accepting responsibility to help and advise the patient as far as he can. Thus when a dying patient appeals to his doctor/friend for help and support he is making greater demands, demands to which the doctor may or may not be willing to respond. The conservative or 'minimalist' response is thus common to most initial encounters of doctors and patients, including the responses of members of other consulting professionals to their clients, e.g. lawyers, social workers and ministers. The 'maximalist' response—of being willing to undertake responsibility for total care—represents for many a vocational ideal, but an ideal which frequently cannot be met in practice. Consequently it is more important to explore the characteristics and limitations of the more typical minimalist approach.

The main features of the 'minimalist' view of medical or professional intervention were characterised as follows : i) The doctor or professional contracts to do the thing he can do expertly ; ii) The consulting professional is responsive to expressed needs and does not seek out undeclared dependency ; iii) The minimalist position protects the professional from excessive demands, keeps decision-making within the area of his professional competence and inhibits him from playing God ; iv) The minimalist position respects the independence of the patient/client and protects him from unsolicited and excessive investigation. (E.g. a minimalist approach avoids the danger of over-medicalisation.)

The main objections to the minimalist position were :

i) While seeking to prevent professionals from 'trespassing' outside their areas of professional competence, it also limits their willingness to explore areas of possible joint action. It actually tends to inhibit inter- and intra-professional co-operation and thus in practice reinforces the dominant position of the controlling professional —whether doctor or social worker etc.

ii) It is ideally suited to the professional in the consulting role. It is less appropriate to the role of the 'family doctor', or to operation of the multi-disciplinary Primary Care, Geriatric or Psychiatric team, where the resources of the family and the community need to be mobilised.

iii) Strictly interpreted it serves the interests of the professional more than those of the patient or elient. It safeguards the professional from becoming too involved, but it also tends to limit investigation to the expressed needs or presenting symptoms. The client's right to information tends to be limited accordingly, thus limiting his ability to make responsible decisions or make the best use of available resources.

iv) While seeking to safeguard the rights of the individual it is not responsive to the fact that a marital crisis, mental breakdown or impending death affects and involves others and impinges on their rights. Some compromise on the rights of the patient may be necessary in his own best interests.

Contract, Code Covenant

The question of the nature of doctor/patient or professional/client 'contracts' is not merely a theoretical issue either. The way these 'contracts' are viewed has far-reaching repercussions for patient care and good working relationships. The negotiation of contracts in health-care has traditionally not been a formal or explicit exercise, and the question can be raised whether it is not desirable that there should be more definite consultation, sharing of information and joint agreement in decisions relating to management and treatment.

The significance of the debate about the definition of doctor/patient or professional/client relationships is not in the choice of one term rather than another, but because different presuppositions —different attitudes and values—underlie these different conceptions of relationships. They embody different concepts of the nature and dignity of persons—as professional *codes* tend to treat clients as dependents, *contracts* emphasise their equality and *covenants* emphasise the transcendent ideals of vocation and the dignity of persons involved in relationships of caring rather than the provision of technical services between 'functionaries' and 'consumers'. The different models suggest different conceptions of disease and 'the sick role' or 'dying role'. The choice of one model rather than another is an expression of how the professional views his own responsibilities to his patient and his professional body as well as the question of his accountability to the public. Professional organisations based on Codes have different modes of ensuring and enforcing discipline from those based on vocation and covenant, or contract. (Cf. Martins, R. 1975 and May, W. 1975.)

The solution of the problems of the possible indefinite expansion of the scope of the doctor's responsibility in the care of the dying and the bereaved might be resolved in three different ways: first by abrogating responsibility for the patient, or by accepting heroic sacrifices are required, or by renegotiating the basis of the contract with the patient or family. Balint suggests that the abrogation of responsibility is effected in practice not by crude 'buck-passing', but by 'collusion in anonymity', i.e. by leaving the question of whose responsibility the patient is unspecified and vague. In practice the patient may be referred on from G.P. to Hospital to Consultant without anyone accepting complete responsibility, or the multidisciplinary team may be used as a device by which individual professionals avoid having the finger of responsibility pointed at them. The acceptance of the need to make heroic sacrifices is usually based on the professional's acceptance of some set of ideals or religious beliefs which motivate him to transcend the functional values of his profession. The value of such individuals is not only to their patients or clients, but in challenging the standards of professional service. The more prosaic way would be to re-negotiate contracts and the limits of confidential relationships in the way demanded by changing circumstances. The very insecurity of Social Work as a recognised profession and the undefined and possibly limitless area of need which Social Work has to serve has meant that Social Workers have been recommended to carefully negotiate specific and limited contracts with their clients. (CCETSW No. 13, 1976.)

The 'new' situation created by a fatal prognosis and the limitations this places on what doctors, nurses and others can do, as well as the opportunities the situation opens up for the disclosure of unlimited needs, suggests that the revision and 're-negotiation' of 'contracts' in such situations may well be in the best interests of patients and carers alike.

The 'ethics of intervention' are then the subtle questions of defining the scope and limitations to patients' rights and duties and professional privileges and obligations in a changing situation in patient care. The pronouncement of a 'sentence of death' on a patient may well create acute dilemmas in terms of existing 'contracts' and may demand review and creative innovation in new relationships based perhaps on other models. Like all moral dilemmas, in this case involving conflicts between the value-presuppositions of the old relationship and the value demands of the new terminal situation, these cannot be resolved in principle but can only be resolved in practice by neglect or avoidance or courageous innovation.

SUGGESTED READING FOR CHAPTER FOUR

The studies listed in the Bibliography under Balint (1957/74), Central Council (1976), Cartwright (1973), Freidson (1975), Glaser (1968), Masters (1975), May (1975), Raven (1975), Saunders (1976).

FIVE

Patients' Rights in Terminal Care

IN CHAPTER TWO three issues relating to the rights of the dying were identified : the patient's right to a good death ; whether he has a right to choose how, when and where to die ; what priority should be given to the rights of the dying patient over those of the family or of doctors and other professionals.

The case considered in this chapter concerns a woman, who earnestly wished to die at home but was prevented from doing so because of family conflict which made it difficult for her daughter to nurse her ; because inadequate professional assistance was given to the family ; and because the GP considered that her pain and nausea could be better controlled in hospital.

Current fashionable talk about patients' 'rights' may be unhelpful for several reasons : first, lack of clarity about what rights are as distinct from mere liberties, and consequent lack of agreement about the fundamental rights of patients ; second, unawareness by the majority of patients of their rights, third, because circumstances tend to limit the extent to which people may in fact exercise them. In reality people's rights are best respected by attempts to achieve the best possible terminal care compatible with the circumstances rather than by pious moral talk about rights in the abstract.

An attempt was made to clarify what is meant by 'rights', in particular *the right to privacy, the right to know* and *the right to treatment*. (The question of the alleged right to die is taken up in the next chapter in the discussion of suicide and euthanasia.)

What are the rights of the dying patient?

The National Health Service is built on assumptions about the rights of people to adequate health-care. There appears to be a consensus that patients have certain rights. There may be philosophical debate about whether people do indeed have rights, in the inalienable sense, or whether they acquire their so-called rights only by custom and convention, but there can be little doubt that in Britain there is general agreement that people do enjoy certain fundamental moral, legal and political rights.

Does the fact that a patient is dying make any difference to his rights, and do the dying acquire additional rights which they do not have as ordinary patients? The rights of dying patients are no different from those of other patients, except that the dying patient may have a greater claim on our attention. We owe it to him to respect his rights and to enable him to exercise them as fully as possible, on compassionate rather than metaphysical grounds.

The frequently mentioned right of a patient *to a good death* was seen as a practical extension of his rights into the terminal context. The right *to privacy*, on which the patient bases his expectation that caring professionals will respect his dignity and personal confidences, becomes, as he nears death, the basis for concern how to achieve the co-operation of the family and other professionals without compromising confidentiality, and how to ensure 'death with dignity'. The right *to know*, on which the patient bases his confidence that he will be kept adequately informed about his condition and treatment, becomes the basis of the question of how to communicate the truth and share decisions about terminal care with the patient, and how to respect the requirements for obtaining informed consent. The right *to treatment*, the confidence that the health-care team will do the best they can for him, becomes a question of how far the patient expects attempts to be made to save his life, of respect for the patient's right to refuse treatment, and the responsibility of the professionals to provide the best possible standard of terminal care.

The *right to privacy* is central to the whole question of communication with the dying, including the patient's right to be heard and to have his beliefs and opinions respected. Because the dying patient may be anxious to talk about his personal, financial, moral or spiritual problems, the caring professional to whom he speaks not only has the obligation to respect his confidences, but also to refrain from imposing his own views. Because the moral or religious views of professionals may differ from those of the patient, they should listen sympathetically and encourage the patient to find his own answers, or seek appropriate advice and help from others, rather than attempt to offer unsolicited moral and religious advice of their own.

The importance of *the right to know* was stressed, and there was general endorsement for a policy of openness. In some circumstances the doctor may be justified in withholding the truth from the patient, and is never justified in forcing the truth on him if he is unwilling or unable to talk about it, nevertheless in most cases the patient's right to know should be respected and he should be informed where possible of the reasons for changes in management. The responsibility of the caring professional to share with a patient the truth about his condition also commits him to give the patient appropriate support while he comes to terms with his condition.

The *right to treatment* (or to refuse it) raises difficult questions. Interpreted too narrowly it seems to oblige the health-care team to maintain life for as long as possible without regard to its quality. The professionals have the responsibility to interpret 'treatment' in terms of what is in the best interests of the patient, and this may mean deciding 'to settle for comfort'—itself a proper form of medical care or treatment—when the terminal stage is reached. The patient's right to refuse treatment can create painful dilemmas if interpreted absolutely. Professionals may have to persist with treatment in certain circumstances if the patient is not thought competent to decide. The right to treatment and to refuse treatment cannot be interpreted as absolutes, as treatment depends on the judgment, knowledge and experience of others whose right to decide is also at stake in so far as they may face charges of professional negligence if they make wrong decisions.

It was generally assumed that no rights are absolute because all rights impose corresponding responsibilities on others. The rights of the dying were recognised to be very important, but they may be given undue importance in relation to those of others. The dying may acquire great power over the living, by exploiting the fact that they are dying to make unfair or unreasonable demands on their families or professionals, or by threatening to alter their wills unless their wishes are met. It was questioned whether the dying ought to have this power; professionals may sometimes have to uphold the rights of the family against those of the dying patient where, for example, the patient demands to be nursed only by a particular person or demands the right to die at home when this cannot reasonably be arranged. While professionals should show respect for the dead and the feelings of relatives, there may be circumstances where it is their responsibility to remind the family or the bereaved that the rights and authority of the dead are not unlimited.

The right to a good death has been interpreted to mean not only that the dying patient has a right to the best available form of terminal care, but also that the patient has a right to choose to die, to elect voluntary euthanasia. There was marked divergence of opinion on this subject, but it was not directly discussed in this case-conference.

67

Case presentation

The extent to which the rights of the dying patient are recognised and respected depends on many factors. The freedom of the patient to exercise his rights may depend on the extent to which he is aware of them, and willing to assert them, on the attitude of his family, and the reactions of doctors, nurses and other professionals.

'Mrs Macdonald'

District Nurse. Request to visit woman of 60 with extensive cancerous sloughing tumour of the left breast. Patient had right mastectomy four years earlier. Cross involvement of lymph glands. Treatment ordered:—Dressings by District Nurse and sedation when necessary. No pain, but severe nausea and severe odour.

Family unit : Husband—long-distance lorry driver. Married daughter with young family living in the same road. Married son with pregnant wife living 200 miles away.

The patient knew about her condition but did not want the husband to know, as it would have 'ruined his job' and they needed the money. Services were brought in, such as home help and meals. The latter had to be discontinued because of the nausea. The home help left because she could not cope with the smell and probably because the whole situation upset her.

Hospital care was offered but the patient pleaded to stay at home insisting that she would not be any trouble. The daughter who lived nearby spent a great deal of time with her mother but was worried about the toddler who had to be brought as well, as the child insisted on climbing on 'Nanny's bed'. The son-in-law was helpful and polite to the patient but attempted to persuade his wife to spend less time with her mother so that she would have to go into hospital. On one occasion they had a serious argument about it and the daughter wept when the district nurse arrived.

The patient was totally *compos mentis* and composed. She said that she just longed to live to see her son's new baby—another eight weeks to wait—and she was afraid she would not survive that long in hospital. She had obviously always been devoted to her son, who was the younger of her two children, and she had been heart-broken when he and his wife had moved away. The son came to visit his mother and asked if she could be moved to stay with them. This could not be arranged, because the patient was too ill, because the husband would not have been able to visit, and because the daughter claimed that she was managing

68

all right and she would feel unhappy if her mother went away.

It was decided to leave the patient where she was. The district nurse visited three times a day ; family savings were used to obtain private domestic help. The Marie Curie Foundation provided a night nursing service. The patient deteriorated rapidly ; she could not take any food other than Complan. She refused sedation because she felt it would 'finish her off sooner' and she wanted to be 'with it' when her husband came home.

After four weeks she developed severe pain and nausea. The GP decided that the situation could no longer be controlled at home and it was decided to admit her to hospital.

Hospital Consultant. Shortly after admission to hospital Mrs MacDonald developed steadily increasing difficulty in swallowing, complete loss of voice, and some confusion. The diagnosis was not clear—query stroke, query cerebral secondaries. Noninvasive intra-cranial investigation was commenced and a nasogastric tube was inserted for ingestion of food and drugs.

Several days later the patient developed a right hemiplegia. She became more confused and also became incontinent of urine. After consultation with the neurologists it was decided to abandon intracranial investigations and the problem then became one of terminal care. Her relatives visited constantly but she could not communicate. The staff believed that she knew what was going on and understood what was said to her. The intranasal tube was kept in place for nutrition and drug therapy, but this distressed her considerably, and she was frequently in tears. As the skin began to suffer an indwelling catheter was inserted. The patient developed considerable restlessness and, as far as the staff could judge, increasing distress. It was decided to give her Heroin and Brompton Mixture (Morphine/Cocaine/Alcohol). Her restlessness diminished and she eventually became inert. Possibly due to her inertia she developed a terminal bronchopneumonia and died three weeks after admission.

Comment by District Nurse. The woman's death left a distressed and guilt-stricken family, especially the husband who blamed everybody including the professionals for letting her go. He said he knew she was very ill but thought his wife would suspect something terrible if he changed his job. Ironically some of the difficulties of the situation were caused by the woman exercising her right to keep her secret.

The fact that the husband and wife did not discuss the situation frankly isolated them from one another with resulting complications in bereavement. The whole 'conspiracy of silence' around the patient, a kind of game of 'hide and seek' led to confusion over the management of the patient and aggravated family conflict. The lack of openness meant that less than justice was done to the rights and interests of all parties involved, and the family remained in ignorance of help from social services to which they were entitled.

The task of coping with the network of difficult relationships was left to the district nurse. The GP's minimalist ethic conflicted with the demands of the situation which required further consultation with family members. When he did intervene it was on behalf of the family rather than the patient, so he acted in a way that was inconsistent with the minimalist position which confines itself to the patient's interest. The GP's ethic conflicted with the District Nurse's commitment to total care, and in the absence of a recognised team framework within which responsibilities could be delegated and shared there was bound to be misunderstanding.

The rights of the patient and others involved, including the husband, were not adequately respected, in so far as there was inadequate consultation of all concerned. Equal access to information is essential for the resolution of the practical dilemmas of care. The right of the patient and significant others to share in decisions relating to the management of the terminal situation can only be met if they are given adequate information and assistance to get the benefit of available services.

Comment by Hospital Consultant. In the hospital context there were two phases in the management of the patient—the first governed by therapeutic optimism, the second by the recognition of the situation as terminal. The first phase still involved investigation, diagnosis and treatment, and attempts at rehabilitation. The hope of survival was implicit and there was still a fairly explicit contract with the doctor, to treat what was treatable and that the patient accept some discomfort as necessary. In the second phase the therapeutic prospects were nil. The management changed as survival was no longer the prime concern. The comfort of the patient became the prime concern. The point at which direction changes is decided on technical grounds by the clinical team—when the balance of interest on therapeutic investment changes to a negative quantity. The doctor/patient contract becomes less specific: on the one hand the doctor falls back on the basic requirements of his professional code, but on the other hand may well enter into a more personal relationship (covenant) with the patient (assuring the patient that he will stand by him to the end).

This more informal relationship makes possible a flexible approach to the care of the dying patient. There is scope for other members of the team to accept a greater share of responsibility. Purely nursing functions assume a greater significance and the social worker's or minister's roles may become more important. Good inter-professional co-operation in terminal care presupposes a form of consensus management rather than reliance on the sole authority of the doctor. However, the ambiguities inherent in the less explicit contractual relationship may create difficulties. There may be difficulty in knowing the proper limits of communication with the patient and family. The roles of the doctor, nurse, social worker and others involved become blurred. There may be a tendency to withdraw or 'pass the buck'. It becomes less clear how the rights of all parties are to be safeguarded—how patients' wishes are to be respected, and how professionals are to be protected from unreasonable demands and allowed scope for the exercise of their proper authority.

'With whom is it appropriate to consult on the direction the case is taking? Relations with relatives may be difficult. Patients may not be "all there". Does the doctor convince himself that the patient is unable to contribute and rely on his own judgment or consult with the relatives? Or does he say to the relatives "*I'm* his doctor" and withdraw? Is further consultation with the doctor inhibited by the panoply of medicine, the presumption of the rightness and moral good of the doctor? Or is this belief essential to the trust which the person needs as a patient in distress? If the doctor says it is right and good the patient tends to accept it. We believe it is unfair to put the burden of decision on the relatives, and that it is unfair to involve the patient. They agree with us, they accept our decisions—perhaps because the relatives have become already prematurely bereaved, isolated by the rupture of a relationship. In summary: there is talk of consultation, whereas in reality someone (the doctor?) has to decide between the protraction of an uncomfortable life and settling for comfort—where it is necessary to accept that some consequences of "comfort" will hasten the death of the patient.'

Illustrative Discussion

Dying at home. It was strongly contended that, given the opportunity to choose and the reassurance that adequate help will be given, most dying patients and their families prefer that death should take place at home. Therefore, the supervision of terminal care in the home by a properly trained Primary Medical Care Team

(PMCT) is probably the best way of doing justice to the rights an interests of the patient and his family.

GP. We are developing an institutionalisation of the pattern of terminal care. Patients have expectations of what can and can't be managed at home. There is an assumption that 'terminal' means 'hospital', but we needn't agree. People are happy to explore the possibility of getting things done at home. However this presupposes that an end-point of home management is defined in consultation with all involved and that the resources of the PMCT are effectively mobilised to provide necessary support.

The assumption that terminal care in hospital is more effective and efficient was questioned on both human and economic grounds

SW. Hospitalisation may create as many problems as it solves. In human terms the cost can be very high in isolating the dying from their relatives, with resultant complications in bereavement. The cost of relieving the family of the burdens of terminal care by hospitalisation may in economic terms not be significantly different from supervised and assisted terminal care in the home. The proper use of a Primary Care Team may prove a more cost-effective means of mobilising the knowledge, expertise and resources of society to help the dying, especially if we take into account the human cost of the alternative.

The proper functioning of the PMCT in the home requires changes in the presuppositions governing traditional professional roles, and a more actively interventionist approach if the co-operation of the patient and family is to be secured. The tendency of each professional to start from a minimalist view of his contract with the patient and to retreat back into it when confronted with conflict in the family or disagreements within the PMCT, hinders effective home-care, and drives towards hospitalisation as a possible solution to the difficulties involved. The care of the dying in the home requires a more flexible view of confidentiality—both with respect to the relatives involved, and between different members of the PMCT who share responsibility for the care of the patient and family. Changes in the management of the patient may call for explicit re-negotiation of the implicit contracts between the professionals and those involved. For example, the nature and scope of individual rights needs to be openly discussed, practical alternatives need to be clearly presented, information and decision-making needs to be shared so far as possible, the determination of priorities and choice of available resources should be based on the widest possible consultation.

Chairman. On the rights of the patient and family—the assumption in home care is of the involvement of other family members or friends. The patient calls in his GP. If the GP decides in favour of home management he presumes on the co-operation of the family. Is he right to do so?

1st GP. The GP's immediate response should be to explore the resources in the home set-up. If this is OK the relatives are automatically involved. I don't see the ambiguity.

Chairman. If the GP adopts a minimalist view of responsibility to and for his patient alone, he would be unlikely to favour home care in the circumstances described, and he would not feel he had a right, for example, to initiate a big family consultation.

DN. The patient could always suggest it, or say no.

Chairman. On what grounds does the PMCT base its contractual relationship with families? The PMCT's view is not minimalist but expansionist.

2nd GP. The situation is a developing one, and we don't know how far we have gone. The expanded responsibility is acceptable to me, but it may not be to others. The Doctor, however, is head of the PMCT, and his attitudes will determine how broadly or narrowly the PMCT regards its responsibilities. The patients and relatives regard us all as responsible professionals. They come to us for advice and not direction. If we go too far or take too much upon ourselves, people have a right to object, and they do. However they are often pleased when we go beyond our strictly therapeutic responsibility.

Responsibility for conflict resolution. A discussion of conflicting interests in a family set-up is often necessary for effective patient-care, and essential if responsible decisions are to be taken which are based on consultation and co-operation. The intervention of the PMCT means that the complex problems involving several parties have to be met face on. Professionals cannot avoid becoming involved, even if only to serve a buffering function between conflicting rights and interests. In such circumstances the DN or SW may become the confidant of the family. Responsibility for decision-making may shift from the Doctor to some other of the team.

Psychiatrist. How were decisions reached by the PMCT in this case? The patient vomited her way into hospital. A case-conference and consultation with the family might have helped, but this pre-supposes that doctors and nurses have the necessary skills for conflict resolution. In general they lack the knowledge and experience. Conflict resolution is difficult. It is basic to work in psychiatry, but the outcome is often uncertain. Therapy is a more certain business than conflict resolution, that is why we tend to avoid getting involved. There is also the feeling that a united front should be preserved by the PMCT, and that militates against frankness. The choice between home or hospital may be a choice between different roles for the professional—therapy or conflict resolution.

GP. I agree. We chicken out of it a bit. It is easier to pass the buck to the hospital.

DN. She had very heavy nursing, and the nausea ought to have been controlled. Was it just an excuse for hospitalisation?

Physician. The GP did as much as he could reasonably be expected to do, and in any case the only effective way of controlling nausea is by sedation, and that complicates the issue by making the patient less consultable than before.

DN. The home help left because of the smell. Could a rotation not have been arranged? The GP could have done more to arrange alternative help. There seems to have been a lack of communication all the way through.

SW. Did conflict hasten the end? Was the nurse really able to cope on her own? Might not a SW have done more to help the patient put up with things and help resolve some of the conflict and communication problems? For example, a SW might have been able to deal with the son-in-law and pave the way for the short-term release of the daughter by arranging for the child to be placed in a day-nursery. A SW might have been able to help arrange a family consultation by acting as a go-between with the family and the PMCT.

DN. In the real world it is more often the health visitor or district nurse who has to deal first-hand with the distress and conflicts in the family.

GP. We all have a responsibility to help in resolving such family conflicts—not just as a matter of respecting the rights of those involved, but in anticipating the care of the bereaved.

Patients' rights in hospital. The safeguarding of the rights of the dying patient is more difficult in hospital. The signing of consent forms and admission procedures may mean that the contractual relationships are made more explicit and patients' rights are respected in theory, but in practice there is less room for the patient to exercise them, less opportunity for him or the doctor to renegotiate the limits of their 'contract'. Hospital medicine is more strictly organised—in the interests of efficiency and for the more scientific study and control of disease. The artificial control of the patient and his environment may well lead to a restriction of the rights of the patient and the family. Patients are more helpless—risk loss of

privacy and dignity. Access may be severely limited through restricted visiting and patients may be put under pressure to remain in
hospital and accept further investigation or treatment when they
wish to leave. The theoretical freedom of patients is restricted in
practice by the willingness of doctors and hospital staff to take their
requests seriously.

GP. Admission to hospital should be decided by what is in the
patient's best interests.

Chairman. But hospital admission may be decided by the fact
that the family can't cope. Do the rights and interests of the
family not sometimes come first? It is paradoxical to say that
admission to hospital is 'in the patient's best interest', when the
patient's rights and freedom are likely to be more circumscribed.

GP. I'll rephrase that. Are not the central problems those of the
patient, with the problems of the family secondary to them?
What happens when the family becomes the bigger problem?
Surely the patient comes first?

Ward Sister. But it doesn't follow that hospital is the best
choice. Hospital is abrupt, practical and 'easy' from our point of
view, and may be helpful to the relatives, but it may be distressing to the patient. To witness the distress of the non-com-
municating patient crying helplessly, makes one wonder if they
would not be better off at home whatever the circumstances.

DN. In this case the G P was probably right to hospitalise the
patient because he was avoiding the break-up of the family. The
D N did not see the wider scene. But doctors are too reluctant to
give a prognosis which will help people decide.

Chairman. This highlights the centre of this case : that the G P
was safeguarding the rights of the larger family at the expense of
the patient's rights. His was a gut reaction rather than a rational
moral judgment. This case is the reverse of 'Mr McIntosh', where
it was the patient's rights at the expense of the family's.

Physician. I disagree. The rights of the family are most visible
at home. Family pressure is most influential. Hospitalisation
alters the moral basis, by restoring the one-to-one relation between
patient and professional, with the family being kept more in the
background.

Social Worker. In the institution, the institution takes over.
The individual is more helpless, the professionals have more
authority. The patient's rights are restricted and in practice this
serves the interests of the family.

Ward Sister. Hospital is tidier rather than easier for the family.
You get a sudden gathering of the clan and conflicts may arise. In
hospital at least you can get rid of them. The sister may get quite

pink-cheeked and bustle about to get them out of the way. The staff too can always find someone to hide behind : 'I must see sister', or 'I must speak to the doctor'.

Social Worker. The fact is that the relatives need only take strictly limited doses of uncomfortable suffering when the patient is in hospital. Society interposes professional management and offers total care at the expense of the diminution of the patient's rights—especially the rights to privacy and self-determination. The whole basis of the contract with the patient changes, but is not properly re-negotiated. The signing of consent forms does not safeguard the rights of the patient so much as protect the hospital from liability.

Physician. The family tend to restrict the rights of the patient to self-determination, and the hospital may restore these to some extent, although privacy may be lost.

Chairman. We need to examine the pre-supposition that individuals as individuals have rights. Do individuals as such have rights, or only in a social context where their rights are limited and circumscribed by the rights of others? In some circumstances it may not be possible to meet the demands of the dying patient. Their rights are not ignored but cannot be met without imposing intolerable hardships on others who have to care for them.

GP. The timing is important. When a patient is ambulant, lucid and able to act independently there is a case for upholding his autonomy even at the expense of the rights of others involved. When a patient is bedfast, incontinent and completely dependent on the help of others it is a different issue. If we acknowledge that the patient has rights then we have an obligation to provide what help and services are necessary, including hospital.

Nurse. I suspect that this woman had always been the manager in the family, so that when she became ill the family couldn't cope. Had she always run things, but couldn't run this? Were the family hoping the hospital would take over for the mother? Her insistence on her rights may have been a last attempt to manage the situation her way.

SW. It may have been possible with more adequate resources and by making use of the expertise of other professionals to persuade the family that hospitalisation was not the best solution for them or the patient. The only way that justice could have been done to the rights of all parties involved would have been to have a full consultation of all involved.

DN. There was a conflict in the patient's desires . . . she wanted to die at home but she also wanted to live long enough to see the new baby. This raised a practical dilemma—was it possible for

both the patient's wishes to be met at home? Which was the
more important? Patients' rights have to be considered in terms
of what is practicable. There was even the problem of whether
there was enough time for consultation, resolution of conflicts
and the making of the necessary decisions.

In the end the dying patient is helpless, and depends on others to
enable him to have a good death. In any particular case the extent
to which the patient's right to a good death is respected will be
reflected in the quality of care provided—within the limits of
what is available and feasible. In practice patients' rights will
mean different things in different contexts and will depend for
their interpretation and implementation on the understanding and
compassion of individuals and the skill and proficiency of their
service—whether it be in the home, the hospice or the hospital.
In general the rights of all people to a good death can be secured
only by improving the standards of terminal care. Those involved
in terminal care need to be more adequately trained. Acquisition of
the necessary medical skills should not be at the expense of
other human skills required—the ability to empathise with the
dying patient and to understand his emotional reactions to
dying, to deal with conflict resolution in the family situation, to
learn to work with other professionals, and to cope with the
increased moral responsibility associated with care of the dying.
In summary, the rights of the dying are as real as respect and
compassion permit them to be. The job of the professional is as
much as anything to facilitate others in the realisation of their rights.
Disagreements about rights considered in the abstract become less
important than the consensus worked out in practice in a given
case. The 'best' situation will always be one where justice is done to
the rights of all involved—patient, family and professionals. The
fact that dying is the last experience of life lends it extraordinary
poignancy and importance. The need for professionals to be sensitive to this fact is the most vital part of their moral education rather
than theoretical instruction in the philosophy of rights. The patient's
appeal to his rights, like the suicide gesture, is more often than not
an appeal for help, an appeal for someone to listen, an appeal to be
taken seriously. The dying are less concerned about the philosophical validity of their claim to have rights than with the practical
care and human understanding which enables them to die in peace
and die in dignity.

Analysis of conclusions
While we have taken it for granted that people have moral and legal

rights, the rights that exist in our society may not be acknowledged in other societies. Human rights cannot just be taken for granted even in our own society. Dying patients have a right to special consideration, but in practice the extent to which the dying are allowed to exercise their rights depends on circumstances and the attitudes of other people. Rights have to be fought for and only become established in common law and moral practice by the force of public opinion and by consensus in public debate. The rational grounds for moral rights in general and the rights of terminal patients need to be explored in theory and in practice. Philosophical argument is not irrelevant to the process whereby rights become clearly articulated, but whether they become established in practice depends on the willingness of people to accept the reforms and safeguards which are necessary to protect people's rights.

When someone seeks the backing of the courts for their right to proper medical treatment on the NHS or for compensation in a case of alleged negligent treatment or injury suffered, the appeal for justice is made in terms of the existing rules, and where the assumption can be made that the rules are universally applicable. Appeals by relatives for a court order to restrain a doctor from further treatment of a dying patient, or to prevent him terminating treatment to a seriously ill patient, would involve serious debate about the acknowledged rights of the patient to proper treatment, and the corresponding right of the doctor to exercise his clinical judgment in decisions relating to treatment. The patient's right to privacy, the right to be kept adequately informed about diagnosis and treatment, and the right to treatment itself, as well as the doctor's right to clinical autonomy and the right to refuse to take on a patient follow directly from the nature of their original contract. The presuppositions of the one-to-one confidential and therapeutic relationship are that both doctor and patient have rights and corresponding responsibilities. The patient has the responsibility to be truthful, to give appropriate consent and to co-operate in such investigations and treatment as may be necessary. He has a right to expect that the doctor will respect his right to refuse treatment. The doctor has the responsibility to observe strict confidentiality, to obtain informed consent, and to give medical treatment which is in the best interests of the patient. He has the right to expect that the patient will respect his medical judgment and right to withdraw if necessary.

These corresponding rights and responsibilities are not only generally acknowledged in medical practice, but are sanctioned *in law*. It is possible for a patient to sue for breach of confidentiality, for not having been properly informed about the possible consequences of treatment, and for negligent or incompetent treatment resulting in injury. The courts too are likely to uphold the doctor's right to clinical autonomy.

If appeals to rights are serious and not simply rhetorical gestures, their commonest function is to draw attention to felt injustices. The appeal to 'the Patient's right to a good death' is an example of a situation where on the one hand it is felt that the general standards of terminal care are deplorably low and where on the other there is not yet a generally acknowledged right of the dying to the best possible standard of terminal care. The appeal made in this context to the language of rights represents an attempt to draw attention to the needs of terminal patients, the poor quality of care they receive and the injustice they suffer as a result. The debate about the 'rights of the dying' and the 'right to a good death' which has been initiated by the work of people like Cecily Saunders and Elizabeth Kubler-Ross has challenged the accepted standards of medical and nursing practice and the assumptions underlying the treatment of the dying. To initiate such a debate has at least three purposes—to expand the notion of what patients' rights are in the context of terminal care, to attempt to reform existing institutions and practices, and to re-define the roles and values of health-care professionals in relation to the dying.

To provoke a debate about rights may also be used in the attempt to extend the existing legal or moral rights of health-care professionals, or in the attempt to redefine the priorities of the National Health Service. When doctors or other health-care professionals, for example, claim the right to strike they not only seek to draw attention to their grievances in a way that they hope will achieve for them better pay and working conditions, but they are implicitly redefining their roles and re-negotiating the legal and moral basis of their contract with the patient public. The debate about patients' rights, given the acknowledged obligation of the State to provide adequate health-care for the whole society, will obviously lead to arguments about the scope of the State's obligations and the extent of people's rights—for example, to provide hospices for the dying or more and better high technology medicine, and whether people are entitled to euthanasia on demand, or 'free' drugs, contraceptive aids and false teeth.

Where the campaign for patients' rights is directed towards changing fundamental moral attitudes in society, for example, in the campaign for the 'right' to voluntary euthanasia and the 'right' to abortion on demand, there is a direct clash between opposing sets of moral values. The debate about patients' rights becomes a means to force a re-examination of accepted moral attitudes, or a

79

strategy to introduce moral innovations. Underlying the appeal to the language of rights is the claim that the principles appealed to are universally valid and applicable to all. The clash between opposing sets of values may lead to extreme polarisation in debate rather than any serious attempt to work out a new consensus. Compromise between opposing attitudes to the right to die, for example, may not be possible in principle or in practice. The only solutions which can be achieved in a tolerant society will be ones which seek to remove criminal sanctions from those who conscientiously disagree in theory and practice with prevailing moral attitudes, which seek to safeguard people from being subjected to undue moral pressure from professionals with whom they disagree, and which provide adequate conscience clauses and protection from discrimination for those health-care professionals who do not go along with reformist moral attitudes in their profession or demands from the public.

This is achieved in practice by distinguishing between two kinds of 'rights':—i) rights in the strict sense, where the individual is legally or morally entitled to receive certain benefits or privileges, and where there are corresponding duties on others to assist them to realise their rights; and ii) mere liberties, where the individual is simply allowed to act in a certain way without incurring legal or moral sanctions, and others are under no corresponding obligation to them. For example, with respect to the alleged 'right to die' it is sometimes argued that the legalisation of suicide has created a right to terminate one's own life or have it terminated. These arguments fail to take account of the fact that the English Homicide Act of 1957 and the Suicide Act of 1961, for example, have merely removed the criminal sanctions previously attaching to acts of attempted suicide. Because suicide is no longer a crime, people may be said to enjoy the liberty to take their own lives if they wish to do so. However, having this liberty does not mean that society or the law recognises that the individual has a legal or moral 'right to die', for this 'right' is not legally or morally enforceable, no-one is morally obliged or entitled to assist a person to commit suicide, in fact the law strictly prohibits them from doing so.

In general the fact that in a liberal society certain acts are removed from the sphere of the criminal law, and in that sense become legally permissible, does not mean that they become morally permissible. For an action to be morally permissible (and not just morally excusable in extraordinary circumstances) it must be recognised to be based on universally agreed moral principles. So long as there is disagreement about fundamental moral principles there cannot be valid appeal to 'rights' on the matter, only a rhetorical appeal to others to recognise the existence of rights in an area where they are not yet acknowledged.

SUGGESTED READING FOR CHAPTER FIVE
The studies listed in the Bibliography under Church Information Office (1975), Contact (1972), Cranston (1974), Downie (1971), D'Entrevres (1951), Illich (1975), Kübler-Ross (1970), Marinker (1975), Raphael (1967), Saunders (1967), Voluntary Euthanasia Society (1976), Wilson (1975).

SIX

Is there a Right to Die?

THE CHAPTER CONTAINS two separate but related discussions—a case-based discussion of the question whether one has a right to take one's own life, and a more general discussion of whether euthanasia presents a real moral problem in contemporary medical practice.

Society allows people the liberty to take their own lives, but does not concede that they have a right to do so. Social pressure to treat the suicidal patient as mentally ill implies that doctors and nurses are held responsible for preventing patients from suicide. This view was questioned and the possibility of rational suicide admitted in a limited number of cases. Parallels between custodial care of suicidal patients and care of the terminally ill were observed, including the similarity of the dilemmas faced by professionals if dying patients request assistance to terminate their lives.

The attention currently given to euthanasia arises because there are anxieties (a) about the general standards of terminal care and the indignity of dying, (b) about professionals 'striving officiously' to keep patients alive, (c) about impersonal technological medicine and the helplessness of patients in large institutions. The right of the patient to choose how, when and where to die undermines the clinical autonomy of the doctor, and the existence of such a right was disputed on the grounds that in the therapeutic and caring relationship the rights of the patient have to be qualified by the rights of those who have the responsibility of caring for them. For this reason legal provisions for voluntary euthanasia were thought likely to prove unworkable, but it was argued that except where doctor/patient relations are bad, doctors do co-operate with patients in ensuring their passage to an easy death. Legislation was thought to be inappropriate to the care and understanding which would ensure respect for the rights of patients to have a good death.

The context of current debate about suicide and euthanasia

The central questions are: Does a man have a right to terminate his own life, or a right to expect assistance in the terminating it?

In theory we may argue that people have such-and-such rights. In practice such rights have to be considered in relation to those of other people, to the practical circumstances in which the patient finds himself, and to the responsible professionals involved. The articulation of patients' rights may have normative value—in setting new standards for health-care and changing professional attitudes—but their realisation in practice depends on the co-operation and goodwill of health-care professionals in reforming patterns of institutional care and improving actual standards of patient care.

In the rhetoric of public debate about the 'right to die', in relation to euthanasia and suicide, three issues are raised: the general standards of terminal care; the power and autonomy of professionals (and particularly doctors); and the general policies and ideals governing health-care. In spite of reassurances about improvements in 'death technology' and the professional concern of doctors and nurses to ensure patients a 'good death', there is anxiety that people die in pain and indignity. Doctors may exercise clinical judgment and authority in the best interests of the patient, but there is anxiety that they 'strive officiously to keep alive', that people are kept alive on ventilators as 'living vegetables', that doctors intervene to resuscitate the dying and attempted suicides, that patients are helpless in the large impersonal institution, surrounded by impressive-looking machines. Notwithstanding the ideals of patient-care embodied in the Health Service and attempts to maintain professional standards, there are anxieties about the neglect of the chronically ill, psycho-geriatric patients and the mentally and physically handicapped, and fears that pressure for beds may lead to the covert practice of euthanasia. The anxiety of people to uphold their rights and defend their autonomy in the face of real or imagined professional power and institutional omnipotence, appears to be a most important factor in the debate about the ethics of suicide or euthanasia. These would appear to be the chief conclusions to be drawn from popular support for voluntary euthanasia as evidenced in recent public opinion polls sponsored by the Voluntary Euthanasia Society (see *Guardian*, Oct. 14 1976).

The professionals' response is to emphasise their dilemma—that they are simultaneously responsible to and for the patient on the one hand, and accountable to society and before the law on the other. That society allows people the liberty to take their own lives without incurring criminal sanctions, but does not concede that they have a right do so means that the patient is not entitled to expect assistance to terminate his life. Doctors and other responsible professionals are expected to prevent their patients or clients from committing suicide and are liable to prosecution if they assist someone to commit suicide or in giving euthanasia. As long as there is popular moral repugnance for suicide and euthanasia and an unwillingness to concede that people have a right to die, then health-care professionals have a duty act to protect life and the protagonists of voluntary euthanasia can only continue to try to change public attitudes on the subject. Euthanasia purports to be about the patient's 'right' to have some say in the 'management' of his own death. In its most idealistic form it concerns a man's attempt to make death a significant act, to overcome fate and death as something that happens to him by imposing his own meaning on the event. In reality the facts of human helplessness and need in death, the ordinariness and unheroic character of most deaths, make this philosophical vision somewhat *de trop*. Few people die in the circumstances where such acts of spiritual self-affirmation are possible, and the significance of their actions depends very much on the context and the response of people around them. The person who chooses a religious form of self-affirmation almost by definition, does so in the context of sympathetic co-operation and interactive response with caring persons and this tends to exclude euthanasia as a solution. The patient who insists on his right to voluntary euthanasia faces a paradox: in asserting his right to self-determination he simultaneously surrenders his power of self-determination to another (e.g. the one who administers the last injection)—unless he commits suicide.

A right to suicide?

Moral attitudes to suicide have throughout history been remarkably unanimous. Even the Stoics and certain Existentialist writers who have sought to justify suicide in certain circumstances have condemned it when the action is dictated by cowardice or the fear of death. Seneca, for example, condemned suicide as an act dictated by anxiety: those who 'do not want to live, and do not know how to die' (Tillich, P., *The Courage to Be*, 1952). Seneca argues that suicide is justifiable, as an act of cosmic resignation in which the individual affirms his rationality and the rationality of the universe in the face of overwhelming fate, yet Sartre insists that suicide is absurd—a contradiction of human freedom and rationality. (Sartre, *Being and Nothingness*, 1969). Philosophers like Nietzsche argued that in the right circumstances 'free death' can be an act of consummation and ecstatic self-fulfilment, yet reserve this right to the extraordinary individual. Others like St Augustine have argued that suicide contradicts the basic loves which drive man to live and relate to other people, that suicide is the expression of the derangement of man's loves. In general suicide has been condemned on moral grounds, though often condoned in particular and exceptional circumstances. (See Thompson, I. E., 1976.)

The realities of experiences and medical practice bear little relation to the grand tragic gestures of Stoic or Existentialist philosophers. The studies of 'parasuicide' have shown that the vast majority of attempted suicides are not intended to succeed, but are rather the expression of immediate distress and a 'cry for help' in a situation of crisis. The mounting evidence that parasuicide represents a different class of phenomenon from suicide, and that the overwhelming majority of people who successfully complete suicide are known to have been suffering from serious mental illness, calls in question the picture of the rational suicide as someone who, in full possession of his senses and faculties, asserts his 'right to die' by killing himself. (Stengel, E., 1970.)

Rational suicide remains a possibility, and in a limited number of cases would appear to typify real moral dilemmas. The case considered in this chapter is ambiguous from this point of view, and even the theoretical possibility of rational suicide raises important questions about the extent of patients' right and the limits of professional responsibility.

In practice the debate about euthanasia tends to become a debate about the adequacy of standards of terminal care. Those who advocate voluntary euthanasia are in effect saying that the standards of terminal care are never good enough to prevent some people dying in extreme pain and distress with loss of dignity. The idealisation of man in his freedom, rationality and dignity become the means of attacking and attempting to reform institutions and practices which tend to dehumanise men. To focus attention on the heroic death and the alleged right to die is to some extent to miss the point of this critique.

Case presentation

(This case conference, which originally took place at a Working Group meeting, was published in the *Journal of Medical Ethics*, Vol. 3, No. 2, June 1977. It is reproduced here in a slightly edited and abbreviated form with the kind permission of the Editor.)

'Sybil'

Case history—a Psychiatrist. Sybil was a 27-year-old single girl who had a good science degree from an English university and had been working in a research post for two years before her first contact with psychiatrists following an overdose. This incident was closely related in time to her being offered a position of greater responsibility.

On admission she was thought to have a depressive illness and was treated by a colleague with anti-depressant drugs, and, some weeks later when she showed no response to these, with ECT. She did not change significantly and twice tried to kill herself while in the ward. After four months she was transferred to my care as it was felt she needed more nursing supervision at night which was not available in the first ward. She remained morose, gloomy, and continually confronted those around her with her wish to die. In other respects she was intelligent, quite active and did not show any classical features of depressive psychosis.

She was an only child of academic parents and had lived a rather solitary life at home, even when attending university. Although she had few friends she seemed over the years to be making a superficially-adequate adjustment to life because of her prowess in passing exams. She had had polio as a child and one leg was somewhat deformed. She felt that this rendered her unattractive, particularly to men. She had had no sexual experience.

Her stay in hospital was turbulent and prolonged. She would engage nurses in long discussions about the purpose of life and present her own case for wishing to end it. Many of the nurses who were closest to her found this experience very distressing and regular team discussions usually divided between those who regarded her wish to die as an illness and those who felt it to be the outcome of her particular view of life but not evidence of pathology. This debate was also reflected in those who wished to restrict her freedom by compulsion if necessary and those who believed this to be unjustified. Initially she was under constant observation and made several further serious attempts on her life; although her attitude remained unchanged, the attempts became less frequent and she was given greater independence. She left to live in a hostel after 18 months and attended twice weekly for out-patient psychotherapy. She continued to say she would kill herself but seemed to be coping. She did successfully commit suicide after an out-patient session and was found dead in a friend's flat.

Two months later I received the first of a series of critical letters from Sybil's mother implying that I had 'let this sick girl die'.

The rite of suicide—Philosopher. A case of suicide. Is that the correct ethical diagnosis? Or are we being misled by the presenting symptoms and ignoring the real causes of the doctor's uneasiness? Is it not perhaps the doctor who is the patient in this case—being made to suffer at the hands of the suicidal patient who has wrested the initiative from him? The treatment meted out to the doctor by the suicidal patient leaves him in doubt and uncertainty with all the role confusions and undignified helplessness of a patient. Suicide is an act which calls in question both the medical and moral authority of the doctor. Is this not the reason why the doctor finds the suicide of his patient so disturbing rather than moral doubts about the issue of suicide?

As presented, the case would seem to represent not one single dilemma, but at least three levels of dilemma: theoretical, about the appropriate diagnosis; practical, arising out of the conflict of medical and custodial roles; moral, relating specifically to the issue of suicide.

The doctor's dilemma begins in this case with the absence of an unambiguous diagnosis. He is uncertain about what general principles to apply to the particular case. His helplessness begins with not knowing. However, as Friedson has remarked: 'As a consulting rather than scholarly or scientific profession, medicine is committed to treating rather than merely defining and studying man's ills.'[1] The consequence is that in the situation where no clear-cut diagnosis is possible, the doctor is bound to experience uncertainty and even anxiety. He is caught between the scientific ethic which requires of him that he should have some reasonable theoretical explanation for his intervention, and the medical ethic which urges him to act to alleviate distress.

Given the need to act he is confronted with two different models of psychiatric illness: the clinical/medical model of disease, or the social/custodial model of deviance. He is faced with a choice between different possible therapies based on different theoretical models—as between clinical treatment for organic disorder and psychotherapy for a psychological disorder, and behaviour therapy and social therapy for disturbances of behaviour and social deviance.[2]

At the moral level he is faced with a similar choice of possible roles. To the extent that he responds to the needs of the particular patient and adopts the consultative/medical role, he tends to adopt the individualistic and personal values which go with that role. To the extent that he responds to pressures from the family and society and adopts the custodial/probation officer role he tends to adopt the universalistic and reforming values which are appropriate to social control and behaviour modification.

What does this mean in relation to the patient with suicidal tendencies and no obvious pathology? It means that even before the issue of suicide arises as a moral issue it is viewed within the horizon of other theoretical and practical dilemmas which also have definite moral implications.

87

The shocking thing about suicide is that the suicide is using his death to say something. Whether what he has to say by his death is acceptable to us or not, whether his death condemns us or simply calls in question our authority over his life, can we deny him the right to use his death in this way any more than we can deny the terminally ill the right to make of their dying a significant part of their life? Can we deny to a man or woman the right, by the rite of suicide, to give a final human meaning to a life which has become humanly meaningless?

Our answer will depend on what we mean by 'rights' and to which values we give priority—individualistic values or the common good. Obviously the suicidal or the terminally ill patient has no 'right' to take his own life—in so far as rights imply obligations on others to assist us. The 'right to die' is not enforceable. However, 'the right to die' can mean simply 'having the liberty to'. In that sense the question is: Do we have the right to deprive others of this liberty? This brings us to the question whether it is 'right to commit suicide'. This can either mean, Is it morally right to commit suicide? or Is it morally justifiable to commit suicide?

Even the Stoics, who argued that suicide was morally justifiable if it was the only way a man could affirm his freedom, rationality and emotional detachment in the face of overwhelming, irrational and humiliating circumstances, still insisted that the conquest of the fear of death was the goal and suicide dictated by fear or guilt was dishonourable and disgraceful. The consensus in the moral traditions of the West has been that viewed from the standpoint of the common good, suicide is an evil; that it is an act contrary to reason (Kant); that it is a product of the derangement of a man's loves (Augustine); that it is the result of compulsion not freedom (Sartre), that it contradicts man's social nature (Aristotle, Marx). However, viewed from the standpoint of charity and the desperate need of the individual, it may be morally excusable, even the last essentially human act possible, in an otherwise inhuman situation.

References

(1) Friedson, Eliot. 1975. *Profession of Medicine*, p. 252. Dodd, Mead.
(2) Clare, Anthony. 1976. *Psychiatry in Dissent*. London, Tavistock.

A rational suicide—QC. The normal legal responsibility of a doctor is to take reasonable care to provide advice and treatment, in accordance with reasonable professional standards, to a patient who consults him. The duty probably extends to include the continuance of care or supervision until either the need for any treatment comes to an end or the patient is transferred to the care of another doctor. The doctor's obligations are, however, limited by the fact that the patient has an absolute right to decline treatment. It has long been the law that treatment carried out without the patient's consent, express or implied, amounts to assault. In the case of physical illness in an adult and responsible patient these standards are clear, however difficult it may be to apply the test of reasonableness in a particular instance in practice.

When the patient is not adult or responsible, it becomes more difficult to define the limits of the doctor's duties. It is clear that a doctor presented with an unconscious patient in need of attention is both entitled and obliged to take at least any steps necessary as a matter of emergency. Although the point has never been the subject of a direct decision in court, it is thought that it is probably the doctor's duty to take necessary steps, even if the patient refused treatment so long as he was conscious and able to do so. If the patient is conscious but not capable of taking a rational decision by reason of mental illness or physical weakness, the position is similar. The doctor's obligation is to give the necessary treatment and care to preserve the patient's life even if the patient does not actually wish (so far as he is capable) that that should be done. The obligation extends to a duty to take reasonable care, if necessary by continuous supervision, to prevent a mentally ill and suicidal patient from harming himself.[1] The doctor's duties to a patient who is not responsible thus differ radically from his duties to one who is responsible. The relevant rules are rules of common law and are designed to reflect, and probably do reflect accurately, what people in general expect from a doctor, that he will look after a patient who is unable to look after himself.

I read the account of Sybil's case as indicating that she did not exhibit any signs of mental illness or of inability to take a rational decision other than her persistent determination to end her own life. I also take it that there was no reason to expect that a release from or reduction of supervision would or might have any beneficial effect upon her. If so, the case is sharply distinguished from the more normal case in which the risks of releasing a patient from supervision have to be balanced against possible therapeutic benefits, and the following comment has no applica- to that more normal type of case. In Sybil's case the problem comes to be whether the determination to die in itself is sufficient to show that she was not responsible.

Clearly, such a thing as a rational suicide is conceivable. It would be rational for a man to kill himself to avoid certain death by torture, although no doubt opinions might differ on whether it would be morally right for him to do so. At one time, in English law, the property of a convicted felon was forfeit, and forfeiture could be avoided by suicide before conviction. It might therefore be rational for a man to commit suicide to preserve the benefit of his property for his family. Nevertheless it seems probable that the general and normal reaction is that, in the absence of some clearly defined reason of the sort indicated in these examples, suicide indicates mental disturbance. The popularity of the verdict of suicide while the balance of the mind was disturbed in coroners' inquests was one indication of that view, even though the prevalence of that verdict was in part a result of the fact that suicide ultimately became, in English law, a felony which itself brought forfeiture of property.

In my view, a court considering a case such as this would be likely to reflect this normal reaction. It would not be easy to convince either a judge or a jury that a persistent determination to die, such as Sybil exhibited, was not in itself sufficient evidence that she was not 'responsible'. That is, in effect, to say that a court would be likely to begin by regarding her commitment to ending her life as such a serious limitation of her ability and freedom to manage her own affairs that she should fall into the class of patients who must be looked after. In this particular case, the total absence of any other sign of mental disease might well make it possible to convince a court that Sybil was 'responsible', but the case remains difficult from a legal point of view.

Reference
(1) Selfe *v.* Ilford and District Hospital Management Committee, 1970. 114, *Solicitors' Journal*, 935.

A terminal illness—General Practitioner. We meet Sybil after the first attempt on her life. We do not know how long she had been contemplating this act but the trigger, at least, seemed to be her change in status at work. She was considered to be suffering from depression. This certainly seemed a reasonable diagnosis to start with, and she was treated in a reasonable medical manner. Repeated attempts on her own life might be thought to have confirmed this diagnosis: but in fact her doctors seemed to have changed their minds.

We are not told in detail about her symptoms, but apart from being lugubrious and constantly looking for attention, she apparently showed none of the classical features of depressive psychosis. That Sybil was not helped by anti-depressant treatment, however, does not seem to have influenced her psychiatrists adversely and care was intensified. Everyone was laudably patient with her, but now doubts creep in. If she still insisted on taking her life, but did not have the features of depressive illness, was she mentally ill at all? The question was crucial to the psychiatric team in its discussion, for if she was not mentally disturbed but simply wishing to die, did they have any right to prevent her?

She was presumably detained under one of the sections of the Mental Health Act (1959) '. . . for treatment . . . in the interests of the patient's health or safety'. There was a threat to safety, but if there is no treatment possible, is detention justifiable? Drugs and ECT made no difference. Psychotherapy could hardly consist of more than support in the hope that her attitudes might change. So Sybil was really committed to hospital confinement for, or to, life.

The situation could be redeemed provided that there was a continual attempt to understand her apparently twisted thoughts. Her actions could not be seen as impatient gestures, gambles with life, delusions or manipulative attention seeking—although obviously attention needing. As Camus observed, 'An act such as this is prepared within the silence of the heart, like a great work of art'. So we must know more about Sybil herself.

Her upbringing was hardly a normal one. The crippled only child of academic parents, she had few friends. We know little more but many questions instantly spring to mind. Why an only child? Was the home one of constant tension? Were her parents totally 'unphysical' people? Was she invested with some major unfulfilled hope of their own? Did she lose her father, or anyone else important, when she was young? What was her relationship like with her mother? Why was she always alone? And so on, and so on. From the mists gradually emerges a child, lonely, ugly, infinitely unhappy. Her only prowess was in exams, and her life in no way allowed her physical, emotional or sexual self any satisfaction and fulfilment. Unlike Beatrix Potter, for her there was no Lake District. Her over-compensating, controlling mind, faced with yet another burden which provided no answer to the poverty of her existence, sought solace in death.

If this view of Sybil is anywhere near the truth, she was as 'incurable' as someone with acute leukaemia or terminal chronic bronchitis on a respirator. The end could be put off, but not altered. The physician, while struggling with all his might, must prepare himself and the relatives and help to create a 'good'

91

death. Only when this had been faced could the ethical problem of discharge be considered.

It is not clear that it was, and something does seem to have gone wrong between psychiatrist and mother. It may have been important to keep mother from daughter, but not from psychiatrist. Once it was clear that so little progress was being made, then the mother should have been clearly told of the likely outcome. However little she wanted to hear this, it had to be said, to protect her, to protect the psychiatric team.

Ultimately, as many prison records bear eloquent witness, it is impossible to prevent suicide in a really determined person by custodial means. Medicine has no alternative answers here either. The basis of medicine is to preserve life and health. In some circumstances these two aims may conflict, and although we have made massive advances in our abilities to preserve life, we have not made the same progress in our ability to offer health within that preserved life. Unless doctors point out their limits there is a danger that medicine will be blamed for the things it cannot prevent and will be rejected altogether. There are signs in some quarters that it is happening already, and I think it happened to Sybil's mother.

It was emphasised that the debate about the 'right to die' needs to be rooted in a real context — by being related either to actual cases, or to the actual socio-historical situation in which the question has been raised. Actual decisions are grounded in real situations and even the philosophical debate about whether suicide is morally justifiable has to be seen in its context. To cut out the socio-historical co-ordinates leads to a trivialisation of the challenges of suicide and the demand for a right to die. Two practical approaches were suggested. If we are looking for rules we can take an intellectual approach and consider the range of notions and values worked out in the course of history, but this requires that we recognise, for example, how the Stoic justification of suicide was related to the whole cult of honour in Roman society, dominated as it was by military virtues; and how Existentialist views were related to experiences of men in the Resistance in war-time France. Alternatively we can take a sociological approach and consider: What are the pressures on Doctors? What would a jury accept? What would society tolerate? Either way we are seeking rationalisations for practice in an evolving situation where new technology contributes new definition to the problems of professional practice. We seek by both practical and theoretical means to reconcile ourselves to values.

Euthanasia—Is there a problem?

In a number of earlier discussions when the issue of euthanasia was raised it was fairly unambiguously suggested that the question was not a live moral issue in medicine. There was a tacit assumption that, given the provision of good terminal care, the problem of euthanasia would cease to be a moral dilemma. Likewise the issue of whether the patient has a right to die, tended to be dismissed as hypothetical—for, it was argued, very few people actually claim such a right; and, it was suggested, for someone to want to die might be taken to indicate pre-terminal depression which might be treated successfully with drugs or psychotherapy. To test whether there really was a consensus in the Working Group on these issues it was decided to have a special session devoted to the question. The result was quite marked disagreement.

The surgeon and physician who introduced the discussion both agreed that euthanasia was a pseudo-problem, and maintained that it was basically reducible to a problem of medical management and clinical judgment.

Surgeon. I take the view that euthanasia is a non-problem, that it is not such a real issue in medicine as the public tends to imagine. Only last Saturday I had a patient in my ward—a woman in her late 30s with incurable cancer which had already affected her liver and lungs and was causing her great distress in breathing. I saw her relatives and reassured them that the patient did not have to die a horrible death and that she would be given drugs to prevent her suffering. On Monday she was found to be suffering from severe dyspnoea and was very frightened. She was given diamorphine and died within two hours.

You may call this euthanasia. If so it is euthanasia by necessity. I would call it good medicine. No doctor is willing to prolong life unnecessarily or allow unnecessary suffering. This is not killing but an act of mercy. If controlling the patient's pain and distress means their premature death, this cannot be harmful. The chief ethical problem is whether the patient should be told that the remedies offered will hasten their death. This is a difficult problem to which I don't know the answer. In general the patient is not normally told unless they say they want to know. If they are told, you don't tell them directly that they are going to die, you tell them in a quiet, unhurried and properly edited way that things are not going too well. A patient's anxiety can be relieved by being told. The hastened death may well result in an improvement of the quality of life.

Euthanasia by omission is another kind of situation—i.e. do

we treat a condition knowing that quality of life will be poor? The question here is how hard we should be striving. Should we be treating pneumonia in patients with incurable cancer? The ethical problem rests with the doctor. The moral dilemma tends to be solved by increasing experience and knowledge. The doctor's job is not to keep patients alive at all costs, but to keep them comfortable.

Euthanasia by disconnection is really a non-problem. The disconnection of life-support systems does not involve a decision to kill the patient. One has to decide before-hand if they are alive or dead. The definition of death in terms of brain death has recently been accepted by the Government. The issue becomes one of medical diagnosis, not a moral dilemma.

In all these situations euthanasia is a non-problem. The proper role of the doctor is to strive to maintain the quality of life.

By contrast death by commission is not euthanasia. The positive elimination of 'useless' members of society (e.g. idiots or the senile) is not euthanasia but homicide. There are cases where doctors actively intervene. Some years ago there was a surgeon who if he found fatal carcinoma cut the aorta, and there are cases of nurses who have given fatal injections of insulin to the incurably ill. However, this is not normal medical practice and I am certain it is wrong.

We are left with 'death on demand' which amounts to the demand for 'assisted suicide'. Attitudes to suicide have become much more liberal, but can we condone suicide/homicide on request? I don't believe anyone has the right to demand this of a doctor. If this is a possibility for the future I only hope it doesn't happen. For me it would present no dilemma. I simply wouldn't do it.

Physician. I agree emphatically. Euthanasia never has been a live moral issue so far as the doctor is concerned. Contrary to the evidence of the recent survey by the Voluntary Euthanasia Society, reported in the *Guardian*, October 14, 1976, which suggested that out of a sample of 2,125 people, 33% agreed 'strongly', 36% 'moderately' and only 17% disagreed with voluntary euthanasia, I believe that most of the population would disagree with voluntary euthanasia if they appreciated the full implications of what is proposed. Lord Raglan's bill foundered on the question of what practical guidance to give to doctors. The philosophical issue remains: whether it would ever be right for a doctor to kill a patient even when authorised to do so by the patient. Because of the uncertainty of medical prognosis and the need to involve the patient in the decision there is no possibility of euthanasia on demand being accepted. The fact that the debate about euthanasia continues is due: first, to the poor general standards of terminal care, and second, to the fact of poor doctor-patient communication.

The Incurable Persons Bill did not adequately account for the necessary clinical freedom of doctors. Comprehensive legislation is not possible. Voluntary euthanasia, if permitted, would place intolerable pressures on the clinical judgment of doctors and limit their professional freedom. It would almost certainly put up barriers to good medical practice and make many people reluctant to entrust their lives to doctors.

In this life, life is the most valuable thing we have. It is not to be treated lightly, and early termination is always a lonely and painful decision for the doctor. Sometimes there is no alternative and one can recall such instances as patients with malignant involvement of the pericardium where immediate action became necessary to secure relief from intolerable distress and which could only be achieved by opiates in dosages far in excess of those usually employed. In these contexts comfort is the overriding priority and it is the doctor's primary duty to spare the patient a traumatic end when it is evident that this will be the outcome.

Unless you are a doctor and know death, you cannot know its complexity. This is why so many writings on euthanasia are academic exercises without bearing on the practical reality. Relatives expect doctors to relieve suffering and to give comfort. Only occasionally do relatives or patients plead for something to be done. Usually they are reassured when the pain or distress is controlled. Most current clinical practice is in line with public opinion. The doctor's decision must be an individual opinion in an individual situation, it cannot be dictated by general rules or legislation. The doctor can only offer skill, friendship and perhaps a living faith. His skill is underwritten by his medical training; his friendship is an individual thing and cannot be demanded; his faith may be a means of comfort to the patient—but voluntary euthanasia imposes duties on the doctor which frustrate all three.

The autonomy claimed by the medical profession has to be matched by correspondingly high standards. The standards of medical practice have always to be seen to be high. The activities of the GMC have never been more important. If doctors can be seen to be genuinely responsible and caring people then many of the theoretical objections of the proponents of voluntary euthanasia fall away.

However, it is crucially important that doctors should be seen

to care, and this means that the doctor has to be able to empathise with the patient, the relatives and his colleagues. We must
put ourselves in the patient's place, where we well might be
(Ezekiel: 'I sat where they sat'). If the doctor can fully empathise
with the patient in his unique situation there is rarely disagreement with colleagues about the course of treatment chosen. This
is not 'under-cover euthanasia' but good medical practice.

Illustrative discussion

While there was broad agreement with many of the opinions expressed by the Surgeon and Physician, it was felt that they had
tended to focus attention on the question of the clinical freedom
and responsibility of doctors rather than on the rights of patients.

Chairman. Have we a genuine consensus here? Are the aims of
the Voluntary Euthanasia Society already achieved by good
medical practice? Has the problem been redefined, out of ethics?
Or are there other cases, those of the chronic sick, the unclear
areas, are they different? Has the VES the less clear areas in mind
—areas where doctors are less directly and less dramatically involved? Can the ethical question be reduced to a technical one?'

QC. 'It is difficult for those without the clinical experience to
judge the cases and decisions presented. However, the problem
has probably less to do with the patient about to die than with
the patient living with a fatal diagnosis. At law the cases described
would probably go unquestioned. The situation might be different though in the case of a patient not actually dying, e.g. the
patient with severe anoxic brain damage—where relatives and
carers must be tempted to intervene positively. In such cases legal
and moral dilemmas remain. Further, although the means exist
to control terminal pain and distress, the cases where the means
are not available or are not provided, still raise questions about
the desirability of voluntary euthanasia.

Philosopher. John Wisdom once said: If you want to know
what someone's presuppositions are, look at his examples. The
cases which serve to emphasise the doctor's responsibility and
need for clinical freedom in the management of terminal patients
will not be the same as those which bring out the patient's need
to affim his dignity by asserting his 'right to die' or his right to
some say in the management of his death. The VES case is not
seen from the doctor's point of view, but is about the relationship
of patients to doctors, seen from the patient's point of view. This
may be simply another example of middle-class anticlericalism,
an anti-professional revolt, but we need to ask whether it doesn't
mean more than this? Do people want more say in relation to

their dying? Do people resent that doctors seem to control their lives and 'manage' their dying? Death may be seen, as some philosophers have emphasised, as a crucial moment, a moment for the affirmation of personal dignity through making of one's death a free act. People object i) to being deprived of the knowledge that the end is near, and ii) to having doctors decide what's good for them and prevent participation in the decision. The right to know is the right to discuss these matters. However the doctor's view predominates.

Surgeon. What about the right not to know?'

Chairman. 'Like Ned Seagoon saying: 'I don't want to know that!'

Social Worker. If euthanasia is a non-issue why is there so much anxiety around the subject? Is it because people are wanting to control their own destiny? Because they seem to be asking for help to kill themselves? Why should we find this so disturbing?

2nd Physician. The philosophers' problems will be solved by one practical measure—the ready availability of fatal doses across the counter.

Houseman. They already are available. But that isn't the point. It is about doctor-patient communication in the face of suffering and death.

2nd Physician. I disagree. Would a consensus on the right to die include a willingness to stop standing across the means of a comfortable demise? Why drag people back when they have made up their minds? Why must Doctors be involved?

Philosopher. The doctor *is* involved, because the patient has to rely on information from him concerning his prognosis. If his condition is fatal, has he not a right to ask that his life and suffering will not be prolonged? Does he not have the right to discuss the termination of his life with his doctor?

Registrar. The cases where consultation is a possibility are mainly hypothetical.

2nd Physician. No one has ever asked me that sort of thing. It may reflect the impeccable nature of my practice!

Psychiatrist. Patients say: I'm awfully tired.

2nd Physician. Or 'I've lived long enough'.

Physician. But you don't act on it.

2nd Physician. If they're distressed you treat their distress.

Registrar. 'I've lived long enough' is a comment on quality not quantity of life.

Psychiatrist. The concern with voluntary euthanasia seems to arise chiefly from the anxiety and determination of the living to avoid being trapped in a situation of living death. The images people have in mind are those of chronically degraded patients suffering from dementia or incurable depression, incontinence and extreme physical disability. The fact that many such people exist in psychogeriatric wards and elsewhere is enough to keep the issue alive as a real issue.

Legislation in this area might create more difficulties than it solved. Legislation alone could not guarantee patients' rights or that doctors would act responsibly. The major difficulty would be to establish informed consent. Requests for mercy-killing would be impossibly difficult to negotiate and hence the safeguards required would be so complicated as to make any legislation ineffective. Even if the legalisation of voluntary euthanasia was effected by an enabling act it would still have the effect of creating suspicion in the minds of the public about the intentions and integrity of doctors. It was suggested that legislation of this kind might act as a disincentive to the improvement of standards of terminal care, could lead to the neglect of the study of presently incurable diseases, and by lowering thresholds of caution could lead to wrong clinical judgments. The value of kidney donor cards had proved minimal and similar provision for candidates for voluntary euthanasia was likely to prove useless.

To relieve pain or to kill. Another issue, debated with some feeling, was whether it is possible to distinguish in practice between the intention to relieve suffering and the intention by so doing to terminate a life. The ambiguity of this situation was stressed with doubts being expressed about the 'principle of double effect' being sufficient to exonerate the doctor or nurse when they know that the consequence of their administration of a drug may be the death of the patient.

Chaplain. What is the primary aim in giving diamorphine? If it is given to shorten life then it is morally wrong. Many nurses believe that excessive doses are given, some even that pressure for beds can affect the issue. These are the kinds of suspicions that get around once you talk of euthanasia.

Registrar. ...Some words in praise of heroin. It relieves pain, it relieves anxiety but it also shortens life. Nurses are often anxious not to be the one who gives the last injection.

Chaplain. It is vitally important for the doctor to be clear about his intention as this affects not only the issue of legal responsibility, but affects nurses and junior medical staff who have to implement the treatment regimes.

QC. The law is less interested in intentions than in the

mechanisms of control, who controls what you are going. Did the doctor give the injection or did he instruct the nurse? Anybody can come along and see the dosage. If it depends on intention you can't tell what he had in mind. Controls can be verified. Intentions are impalpable. Patients' fears about euthanasia can be related to uncertainties about doctors' intentions in treatment.

Chaplain. It may sound Jesuitical, but the question of intention is important morally.

Physician. Yes there is a clear clinical distinction between relieving distress when death is a side effect, and giving a drug to terminate life.

Nurse. The question of intention is important to nurses and determines to some extent who gives the last injection. It is acceptable if the intention is to relieve suffering, but shortening life is not incidental. Nurses know this, and there are certain injections which the staff nurse, or sister always gives.

Physician. If our intention is obscure, let us clarify it. But the public leaves it to us.

While there was no general enthusiasm for the legalisation of voluntary euthanasia there was strong criticism of the tendency of doctors to redefine the issue as a matter of medical management so that the ethical issue becomes obscured. This it was contended, is an expression of medical anxiety in the face of patients' demands that they should have some part in controlling their destiny. 'Just as the Rothschild Report led to a response of self-justification on the part of scientists, so what we have heard from the doctors is a re-assertion of their power and their autonomy. Nice arguments about distinctions of motivation are all very well, but they are liable to be seen as verbal camouflage for an assertion of medical authority and disregard for the questions raised about the freedom and dignity of patients and their rights in matters relating to their death. People feel they don't have the power their dignity requires.'

The issue would seem to be that there is a need for the negotiation of a new kind of death contract between doctors and public where patients' rights and dignity, and the right of the doctor to clinical freedom are both respected. There could hardly be consensus on this issue while the attitudes of doctors and those campaigning for patients' rights remain so polarised. The hope of achieving a new understanding would only be possible once the anxiety of doctors to defend their institutional values was moderated to recognise the countervailing force of patients' rights, and once criticisms of doctors were moderated to recognise the degree of dependence which patients will always have on their doctors.

Analysis of conclusions

That a dying patient has a right to a good death would probably be conceded by opponents of voluntary euthanasia on the grounds that it is not euthanasia but simply good medical practice to ensure that the terminally ill die well. Part of the argument hinges on practical questions—for example, whether terminal pain, depression, nausea, incontinence, etc. can be controlled sufficiently for the patient not to suffer distress and loss of dignity. Those that oppose voluntary euthanasia argue that in general these conditions can be adequately controlled. Those who demand that patients should have the right to have their lives terminated if conditions prove intolerable, point to the many cases where terminal care is not adequate and where in particular pain cannot be controlled, or where the patient has lost all dignity and 'becomes a mere vegetable'. On the surface it appears that the argument could be decided by the balance of the empirical evidence—that is, if it could be proved that death with dignity is possible in all cases then the case for voluntary euthanasia would lose its point, and conversely if even in some cases death with dignity is impossible then it would seem that patients must be given the right to choose. It is clearly not just a practical issue and is not decidable on the basis of empirical evidence, for the opponents of voluntary euthanasis will point to the continual efforts which are being made to improve the standards of terminal care, and those advocating voluntary euthanasia will always point to medicine's failures. It is clear at this point that more fundamental issues are involved, though also that the reason why doctors find the debate so disturbing is that it calls in question their competence in terminal care.

At a deeper level the debate about voluntary euthanasia raises fundamental questions about the nature of the doctor-patient relationship, about the scope and limits of the patients' rights in that relationship, and about the scope and limits of the doctor's responsibilities to the patient. Conversely it raises questions about the doctor's rights and the patients' responsibilities.

It is sometimes suggested that since it is no longer a crime in Britain to commit suicide this somehow entails that people have a right to terminate their own lives and perhaps to have them terminated. This argument is unacceptable on two kinds of grounds— —first general and then more specific. In general we do not have or exercise rights in isolation from other people. The very notion of 'rights' entails someone else (even if only God) to recognise those rights, to respect them and thus to admit some responsibility to assist us to fulfil our rights. Rights arise and are exercised therefore

100

in a social context and in a kind of 'contract' with other people. For this reason it is doubtful whether we can ever speak of a right as 'absolute' or 'unconditional'. Every right is defined and circumscribed by the rights of others. In more specific terms, the fact that acts of suicide or attempted suicide are no longer subject to criminal sanctions in Britain means merely that we have the liberty to take our own lives, not that we have a right to do so and even less that we have a right to expect anyone to assist us. The social context in which rights arise means that rights entail concomitant responsibilities, both on the person who claims a right and on the part of others who can be expected to recognise his right. In the case of the intending suicide the claim that someone has a right to commit suicide would entail that others accept that he has that right and might claim that right for themselves. In practice this alleged right is contradicted by an overwhelming social and historical consensus against suicide as morally justifiable except in extraordinary circumstances.

To some extent the argument for voluntary euthanasia rests on the assumption that the situation facing the dying patient is extraordinary. The attempt has not been made to claim a generalised 'right to die' but rather that in specific circumstances such a right should be recognised. The Voluntary Euthanasia Bill of 1969 provided that the patient or prospective patient should be able to sign in advance a statement requesting the termination of his life if it was believed that he was suffering from 'a serious physical illness or impairment reasonably thought in the patient's case to be incurable and expected to cause him severe distress or render him incapable of rational existence'. This draft bill, which sought to make it not illegal for a doctor to comply with such a request, foundered on the question of what specific guidelines doctors should follow in recognising a request for euthanasia as justified in practice. The underlying assumption is that the partial right claimed for the patient has to be exercised within the sphere of the doctor's discretion and subject to his recognition that the circumstances are sufficiently extraordinary to justify his assisting the patient to terminate his life. The circumstances of the doctor-patient relationship which make it necessary to recognise the patient's right to die is circumscribed in practice, also make it virtually impossible to lay down general rules for the administration of euthanasia. Once again the issue is not merely a practical one—of how you provide adequate safeguards against abuse—but also a moral one, i.e. of recognition of the doctor's right to exercise independent clinical judgment and moral responsibility within the boundaries of the confidential doctor-patient relationship.

This does not mean that doctors may not recognise in particular cases that to proceed with further investigations and treatment is useless, and that 'to settle for comfort' may mean that the patient does not live for quite so long. Doctors would argue that they have to make decisions like this all the time, and that to formalise arrangements for voluntary euthanasia is either unnecessary, or would involve unwarranted interference with their clinical freedom. On the one hand they would argue that they do exercise responsible decisions, in their patients' best interests, about the nature and form of their terminal management, and that with few exceptions they do not 'strive officiously to keep alive'. On the other hand, they would wish to reserve the right to take these decisions in their own interests and to safeguard themselves from claims of negligence or impropriety, without the pressure of external legislation.

The claim that the individual has a right to some say in the management of his death would appear to be based in part on an attempt to uphold the dignity, independence and integrity of the individual in circumstances where he is weak, vulnerable and liable to inconsiderate treatment, but it also expresses an 'anti-clerical' feeling against doctors, a resentment of their power and the sometimes (even degrading) way in which they treat or ignore the needs of the dying.

The attempt to restrict the power of doctors and to enhance the power of self-determination of patients, by legislation, faces a paradox: What is required in order that a patient may enjoy the right to die well and with dignity is greater care and trust. Greater care and trust in the therapeutic relationship pre-suppose the freedom of the doctor and patient to interact in such a way that they can show sensitivity and respect for one another's rights and responsibilities. Legislation can formalise the rights and responsibilities involved but it cannot create the inner conditions without which the therapeutic relationship cannot exist. In fact the very existence of legislation may undermine those conditions.

SUGGESTED READING FOR CHAPTER SIX
The studies listed in the Bibliography under (a) *Suicide*: Douglas (1967), Durkheim (1951 and 1952), Sartre (1969), Stengel (1970), Szasz (1971), Thompson (1976), Tillich (1952); (b) *Euthanasia*: Bok (1973), Church Information Office (1975), Contact (1972), Dent, Downing (1969), Dunstan (1972), Fletcher J. F., Glover (1972 and 1977), Gruman (1973), Healy (1956), Incurable Patients Bill (1976), Raglan (1972), Russell (1975), Trowell (1971 and (1973), Twycross (1975), Voluntary Euthanasia Society (1970), Williams (1973), Winget *et al.* (1977).

SEVEN

Conflicts of Conscience and Professional Duty

THE PREVIOUS case-based studies have considered examples of moral conflict and dilemmas relating to: professional intervention in the care of the dying, the rights of dying patients and whether there is a right to die. In this chapter and the following two we examine three issues relating to the exercise of responsibility in institutional contexts: conflicts of conscience and professional duty; inter- and intra-professional responsibility; and the limits of professional responsibility. Each of these is considered with reference to the care of the dying and the bereaved.

The case presented in this chapter was discussed as an example of 'terminal care by investigation'. In spite of the fact that medical and nursing staff recognised that the patient was dying, and that the patient clearly recognised this herself and did not want further tests or operations, the anxiety of the medical staff to diagnose her condition meant that she was subjected to continuing investigation virtually until she died. As such the case was taken to illustrate the dilemma of those who felt on the one hand that it was their professional duty to arrive at a clear diagnosis, and on the other hand that to 'settle for comfort' and good terminal care would be a more appropriate human response to the situation.

The various dilemmas raised by the case centre around the problems and difficulty of decision-making in institutional contexts. The clarification of the distinction between personal responsibility and professional accountability was seen to require an understanding of the differences between personal morality and role-morality and an awareness of how different circumstances impose different demands on individuals, how each individual may simultaneously exercise different roles which are each governed by different rules and subject to judgment by different arbiters.

In discussing the exercise of professional responsibility the following issues were identified as important: the vulnerability of the professional and the need for frankness about the emotional demands of terminal care, and distinction between practical,

103

theoretical and genuine moral dilemmas, the question of practical strategies for dealing with moral dilemmas, the difficulties involved in the exercise of professional responsibility in institutional contexts without power commensurate with the responsibility involved.

Personal moral responsibility and professional accountability

The individual entering professional life may have a well-developed personal sense of responsibility, but in professional practice or in the life of a complex institution he has to learn to accept and exercise more formal kinds. He has to adapt himself to the exercise of responsibility in concert with others and in different kinds of institutional settings where he is answerable to a variety of different people—clients, other professionals and the public. He has to distinguish between personal responsibility and public accountability—between the sense of being *responsible for* what he does freely in the light of his own moral convictions, and the sense of being *responsible to* others for the proper performance of a formal function either acting in his own professional capacity, under orders from a superior, or in concert with other colleagues.

The exercise of responsibility in an institutional setting is of a far higher order of complexity and requires greater maturity and sophistication than in simple inter-personal relations. What is required is an understanding of role-morality, the more impersonal rules which govern the behaviour of professionals (and others) in performing official tasks or public service related to their professional roles. This kind of morality tends to have been neglected in traditional moral philosophy, which has adopted a more individualistic approach and has concentrated attention on the exercise of responsibility in face-to-face interpersonal relationships. What is needed is a complementary analysis which does justice to responsibility and accountability in institutional contexts (Emmet, D., 1968, p. 158).

The distinction between personal conscience and professional duty suggests that the individual simultaneously exercises a number of roles to which different expectations attach, or to which different rules apply. The roles of 'doctor' and 'friend' may be appropriate at different stages in caring for the dying patient. Other situations may give rise to role-conflicts—as when it is unclear whether to continue life-saving attempts or to settle for comfort. The conflict expresses itself as between different sets of responsibilities and rules for action.

Roles and their morality. When we examine decision-making in institutional contexts it is necessary to look closely at roles and their morality. The notion of a role is borrowed from the theatre and refers to a set of actions by which a character can be recognised in repeated performances of the same drama. Nurses, Doctors, Social Workers and Ministers are not just recognised by the different uniforms they wear, but by the different kinds of things they do. In institutional settings, in hospital for example, where an artificial environment is deliberately created, the same kinds of situations tend to recur and standard procedures become established for dealing with various kinds of emergencies or routine functions. Different tasks are allocated to different individuals who, in regularly performing the same task, acquire experience, proficiency and confidence in the performance of that function. Once the roles of the *dramatis personae* become relatively fixed, rules develop to preserve and perpetuate this division of labour. Like the fixed role of a character in a drama, the professional in performing his role is performing actions which are governed by pre-established rules. Roles, both in the sociological and ethical sense, are associated with repeatable patterns of action in social relationships or institutional settings which are rule-governed.

Clear definition of roles is necessary in institutional contexts, both for reasons of efficiency and so that individuals can know the nature and extent of their responsibilities. It is not surprising therefore that people experience anxiety and moral conflict in circumstances where roles and responsibilities are ill-defined. The classic struggle of physicians, surgeons and apothecaries in the nineteenth century to clarify the scope of their respective roles and responsibilities gave rise to most of the content of traditional medical ethics. The similar debates in the nursing profession between hospital nurses, midwives, health visitors and district nurses have not only been concerned with the clearer definition of different professional functions, but have also been the means by which the values of nursing practice have been clarified. More recently the debate between social workers—between those who see social work as a consulting profession based on the model of individual case-work, those who see social workers as agents of social control, and those who see social workers as a pressure group to bring about social reform—has led to various statements on the role and values of social work as a profession.

The critical reappraisal of roles, responsibilities and professional values can be provoked both when professions are in the process of formation (as in the case of Social Work) or when traditional roles are changing (as in the present formation of multi-disciplinary health-care teams). The uncertainty about who is to take decisions in what circumstances, and the resulting problems of communication between professionals charged with different but perhaps

105

overlapping responsibilities, can give rise to moral dilemmas in intra- and inter-professional relationships which are just as acute as those facing the individual when confronted with a personal conflict of roles. While on the surface the conflicts between professionals may have the character of demarcation disputes, underneath these disputes are moral questions and communications problems relating to the values implicit in different roles. As each action aims at some good and that good determines that action's significance, so each professional function has its own value in the division of labour, and it is proficiency in the performance of that function which is the basis of professional pride. The interests and values served by particular functions find their institutional and formal expression in rules.

Rules and their variety. The notion of a professional implies a body of self-regulating individuals who earn their living by the practice of certain knowledge and skills in the interests of other people (their clients), and who accept the responsibility to maintain certain standards among their members. These are standards of knowledge, proficiency, professional integrity and a high level of client consideration. The most general rules applicable to the professions are rules concerned with maintaining such standards and the values they represent. Within the profession the professional tends to place a premium on autonomy, loyalty, conscientiousness, competence and confidentiality. In dealing with clients he tends to emphasise that he exercises his professional function with justice (impartiality and affective neutrality) and truth (informed objective judgment and respect for people's secrets). In addition, the professional tends to restrict his involvement with others to the area of his professional knowledge and competence, and becomes uneasy when required by circumstances to venture beyond this familiar area.

The most obvious kinds of rules in professional life are the formal Codes of Ethics which have either been accepted by tradition like the Hippocratic oath or have been more recently formulated by national and international bodies; the International Council of Nurses' Code of Ethics, and the Royal College of Nursing Code; the British Association of Social Workers' document Values in Social Work and other consultative documents. These codes may serve to define the identity and collective ethos of each profession and have a symbolic function in regulating the aims of professional practice.

Professional codes give little help in dealing with specific moral problems in day-to-day practice. Day-to-day decisions tend to be governed by the collective ethos of a unit, by implicit understanding, and maxims or rules-of-thumb as to the form and manner in which things must be done. The more riskful the procedures involved—as in medicine—the more necessary it is that such 'rules' should exist, but they exist as much to protect the patient/client from abuse or malpractice as to protect the professional from unfair exploitation, to encourage greater confidence between professional and client, and to ensure that the function in which they are both interested will be carried out.

The conflict between the personal moral beliefs of the individual and the various kinds of rules which relate to his different roles, can create areas of uncertainty and acute moral dilemmas—where there is no obvious way of determining which rules should be given priority.

Situations of various kinds. The different kinds of circumstances in which the professional encounters his client and the particular circumstances of the client himself, impose different moral demands. In terminal care, for example, there are obvious and important differences between the roles and responsibility of caring professionals in 'the home' and 'the hospital'. The rights and status of patients and relatives, as well as those of professionals are subtly affected by whether they are 'at home', 'in the consulting room' or 'in hospital'. The rules—what is permissible and what is appropriate—vary considerably from one situation to another. Whether the patient is lucid and ambulant, or bedfast, incontinent and confused, solitary or has family and community support—affects the function and responsibilities of professionals involved.

Further, 'a situation', from the professional's point of view is a complex of facts and circumstances limited or bounded by particular human interests, defined by particular conceptions of 'the problem', viewed in the light of the professionals' attitudes to what is significant. Thus the doctor's view, the social worker's view, the minister's view and the nurse's view may all have elements in common, but are based on different presuppositions about 'what the problem is'. Each professional will see 'the problem' relative to what he can or can't do, ought or ought not to do. To make a moral judgment in a complex situation involving various people performing different roles means not only having a circumspect vision of 'the facts of the whole situation', but also the wisdom to reconcile the conflicting interests and values operating in 'the situation' for each professional.

Arbiters and accountability. Making decisions and exercising moral responsibility in institutional contexts means that the professional must be aware of those to whom he is directly and indirectly accountable. While he is responsible for his patient/client,

107

he is also responsible to him—in the sense that he may be asked to give reasons for his actions and may even be liable to legal sanctions if he fails in his duty. He is also accountable to his peers, his juniors, his superiors, other professionals and the public in different ways. Institutional morality requires a degree of self-consciousness not required in ordinary inter-personal relationships. The individual may feel responsible to his parents, to his family or friends, or to God, but these arbiters do not have the same power to demand accountability or to exact sanctions that his professional arbiters do in institutional life! The arbiters to whom a professional is and feels accountable form an extension of his personal conscience and act as a check on his actions, preventing him from making impulsive or arbitrary decisions, but also limiting his independent initiative. Where problems can be solved by inter- or intra-professional consultations this is fine, but when confronted by real moral dilemmas, the professional may be tempted to abrogate responsibility for taking decisions and to 'pass the buck', or is thrown back on his personal convictions and may 'go it alone'.

Thus the exercise of clinical and moral responsibility in different contexts requires an awareness of several variables which are always present in decision making—the demands of the particular situation and the different ways it is viewed by those who are involved, the various responsibilities entailed by the different roles which the individual is required to exercise, the question of different rules operating in the situation and what priority is to be given to them, and the various kinds of accountability which the individual owes the arbiters of his actions.

The case presented was intended to focus attention on dilemmas for professionals involving a conflict between their defined professional duties and their personal convictions and feelings. Entitled 'Death before Diagnosis: A Case of Clinical Embarrassment', this rather grim story of 'terminal care by investigation' was presented in order to illustrate that in some instances the decision to change the course of management from pre-terminal treatment based on therapeutic optimism to terminal care where you 'settle for comfort' cannot be made on simple technical grounds. The transition from the one to the other in terminal care presupposes a relatively clear-cut diagnosis and confidence about the likely prognosis. Where both are lacking, severe practical and moral dilemmas arise.

Mrs McGrath, aged 79, lived with her equally aged and frail husband. They had one son in Canada. They had managed together without outside help, Mrs McGrath being the stronger of the two. The husband tended to be confused and forgetful and needed the support of his wife. Presented by a medical registrar.

'Mrs McGrath'

28th August: Referred by her GP to the Surgical Out-patient Department. History of loss of appetite, weight loss, pain in left of abdomen. Constipation. Seen by surgeon who finds an abdominal mass 'best investigated by the physicians after admission'.

28th August: Referred to Physicians, and admitted that day. History and findings as above. Provisional diagnosis cancer of stomach or pancreas, or possibly secondary cancer of the liver. Investigations commence: Bloods, barium meal; endoscopy; biopsy of stomach lining; liver scan; ultrasound scan. The mass is still undefined; possibly pancreas, i.e. inoperable, or colonic, i.e. operable, perhaps even benign.

10th Sept.: (The old lady spent the fortnight in puzzled discomfort. She indicated by her enquiries that she assumed her condition was fatal. 'I just want a few weeks for Dad to get used to it,' she said.) Patient's general condition deteriorates. She bebecomes listless, nauseated, and is sometimes in pain. Further barium studies are contemplated. She develops anaemia and renal failure.

12th Sept.: The surgeons visit to review the diagnostic efforts. They feel that only a laparotomy would provide a definite answer. Mrs McGrath is not at present fit for this. They suggest intensive management of her anaemia and renal failure.

14th Sept.: The latter two problems prove difficult and the attempts to solve them are by now rather half-hearted. The patient continues to deteriorate. There is still no diagnosis.

21st Sept.: Terminal care commenced.

23rd Sept.: Patient dies. PM permission granted.

Three kinds of moral dilemmas were seen to have been involved in this case: i) Must the doctor satisfy his professional conscience that he knows the cause of his patient's condition and can offer a clear diagnosis; or does he stop unpleasant investigations in the interests of common humanity even if he is not certain? ii) If he is uncertain of the diagnosis/prognosis does he share his doubts with the patient or is he obliged to be silent until he knows for sure? iii) If the patient is referred to him by other professional colleagues for investigation is his primary responsibility to them or to the patient, even if the latter means refusing to do the investigations asked?

How far to investigate. It was generally maintained that the doctor's peculiar contribution to the care of the sick is to investigate the cause of the distress, to make a diagnosis, and to decide on a course of treatment in the light of knowledge of the likely prognosis. The doctor as doctor has a primary moral obligation to do a certain amount of investigation. If he gives up before he is reasonably sure he fails the patient. The difficulty arises in knowing what it is to be 'reasonably sure' in a given case. While experience may help an element of uncertainty always remains.

GP. Why did the lady go to her GP? She mentioned 'Getting Dad used to it'. Did she really want investigation or simply to get out of the house to allow the old man to get used to being on his own?

Registrar. Yes, this is a reasonable assumption from the tone of the conversation I had with her. 'I'm in to die—don't want too much done—want Dad to get used to the situation.' The whole staff were worried over this case. She knew she was dying, everyone knew.

QC. Although you might have thought this, when should you as a professional have accepted this? There must be some level of investigation otherwise you would not be doing your job properly.

SW. All the woman may have wanted was someone to share the options with. Someone to go home and explain to her husband or advise entry to hospital for investigation. She wanted help with the choices confronting her in that situation.

GP. Is the sw being realistic about alternatives? You must attempt either to cure or to palliate before you decide to do nothing. Investigations are often necessary even if only to determine how to give comfort.

QC. Similar problems are met in other professions. Your training commits you to following certain procedures. All you can do is test and if there is no result test again. To do less than this might be construed as negligence. You are led from one step to another. The question is whether it is worth it or not. The dilemma is where to stop.

Philosopher. There are different imperatives governing the curing and caring roles in this situation. That is the dilemma. The logic of the curing role drives towards further investigation, the logic of the caring role says stop. Professionals can get carried away by the logic of a particular role or function.

Registrar. Medicine thrives on exceptions. We are always looking for patients to snatch from the jaws of death, looking for the possibility of some fatal pathology which mimics some ordinary complaint. By investigations the doctors might have been able to help and if they could have helped they would have been well satisfied.

Chaplain. We'd be in a sorry state if doctors gave up trying. Why else do G P's send 79-year-olds to hospital?'

Registrar. When after 3 weeks there was still no clear prognosis and the patient's condition had deteriorated, attempts on the management of the anaemia and renal failure were half-hearted. She was spared the barium enema. We settled for comfort when it was obvious she was dying. It was not meant to be terminal care by investigation. The dilemma was when to stop trying.

The cure/care dilemmas were seen to be partly a function of ambiguous situations, but partly a function of ambiguities in the role of the doctor. The interdependence of the curing and caring roles makes it difficult for the doctor to decide when to terminate investigations or treatment, and settle for terminal care. On the one hand it was recognised that the logic of the doctor's traditional role commits him to making investigations, seeking a diagnosis and prescribing treatment, on the other hand the doctor could equally well be seen as the trustworthy, sensitive and understanding confidant with whom troubles are shared and who is seen as a source of support and advice in times of need. The accepted image of the doctor as the one who does battle with death, and the rhetoric which supports this, tends to reinforce the feeling that 'something must be done' and 'the obsession with the machismo of getting a diagnosis'.

In his caring and counselling role the doctor needs more confidence in his own intuitions—the feelings which he has in dealing with the particular patient, based on knowledge and experience. He needs to be reasonably sure, and this involves all his acquired knowledge and skill, but he also needs to make a value-judgment as to whether particular clinical investigations are worth it or whether palliative action is better. This need to make value-judgments as well as clinical judgments is a cause of worry; about the desirability of telling the patient and of sending them to hospital for investigation; about how advantageous investigations will be and knowing that decisions are expected of the doctor; about the patient's increased vulnerability to mishandling in hospital in being subjected to unnecessary and unpleasant tests; finally, about uncertainty and the way this undermines confidence and authority.

What do you tell patients? The dilemmas concerning how much the doctor relies on his intuitions rather than scientific knowledge,

111

and how much he shares with his patients, were seen to be related. It was maintained that if a patient came for help, the doctor and staff were obliged to carry on and not give up. The 'contract' with the patient entailed the expectation that the doctor would 'try to find out what's wrong' and 'inform the patient accordingly' (even though he might well be exploring alternative courses of action in the interests of the patient and the preservation of his own professional credibility). On the other hand, in the situation where someone is dying and knows they are dying the doctor may be reluctant to give up his management and clinical role, reluctant to accept the limits of his own power to help. Clearly there is a risk of the doctor giving up too soon, or of carrying on too long. Either way risks are involved, and riskful judgments have to be taken. It was suggested that doctors tend to err on the side of over-zealous investigation and treatment—especially the younger and less experienced.

1st GP. We doctors always assume that we must be diagnosticians, that it is always we who have to take the decisions, whereas people often simply want to express what they already know—that they are dying—and they regard it as a courtesy to the doctor to tell. They may simply want to share this and want nothing further done.

2nd GP. How can you detect this? I couldn't.

1st GP. On occasions the patient indicates that he doesn't want the whole treatment. You can't always diagnose but you can try to be more sensitive to what people actually want.

2nd GP. I don't want to get involved in semantic argument, but diagnosis is a must otherwise you can't be a therapist.

1st GP. But diagnosis includes intuition of feelings.

Registrar. The other registrar would have done nothing. I couldn't simply leave it at that. Different people have different intuitions. To what extent can you rely on intuitions when you get conflicting reactions from different medical staff?

Chaplain. Responses are not based simply on intuition but also on scientific knowledge, clinical investigation and skilled expertise. You use intuition having seen and treated similar cases. The question is whether you had sufficient confidence to act on your own convictions.

Philosopher. If the clinician lacks confidence in his own judgment he can go on for ever seeking more and more certainty. The quest for certainty is interminable. Professionals have to learn to live with some degree of uncertainty.

Registrar. Some senior doctors have this confidence, have a good bedside manner and can put the patient at ease, but in this case there was no one superior around, we were mainly juniors.

If someone could have said: 'Give diamorphine', that would have been a relief.

QC. Someone of authority was needed.

SW. This is just passing the buck, as it seems was the case between GP, surgeon and physician. There was a need to acknowledge a common problem, to share anxiety about the problem. A value judgment was needed as to whether it was all justified. Doing nothing, continuing futile investigations, looking around for a superior authority, all become ways of avoiding the fact that a value-judgment was needed.

Consultant. The risk is that the public accuse you of 'playing God', when you make value-judgments.

It was generally felt that doctors need to be more frank with themselves about how ill-defined and uncertain the 'science' of prognosis is, so as to avoid creating false expectations among patients and deceiving and worrying themselves about the degree of certainty that is possible. This is specially important in hospital because of the helplessness and vulnerability of patients, their susceptibility to control—'Where the patient's answer is elicited by the tone of the doctor—"Do what you think is right, doctor".' The doctor should be willing sometimes to accept the patient's estimate.

While it was considered desirable that doctors should be as frank as possible about likely prognoses, when asked by patients whose condition was likely to be terminal, it was recognised that in many cases this is difficult because it involves changing attitudes to doctors built up over a life-time.

SW. You can't begin at 79. The familiar pattern of a professional/client relationship cannot be suddenly changed. It is a shock for the patient if after 50 years' treatment with the same doctor and that doctor advising, then in the 51st year the doctor asks the patient what he thinks! The patient could be upset in the change of the doctor/patient relationship.

GP. But surprising things do happen at 80 and especially in the context of terminal care. Elderly patients themselves may demand the renegotiation of their 'contract' with the doctor, may demand that their wishes be taken seriously. On the other hand, the doctor might find himself compelled by the traditional dependence of the patient on his professional judgment to carry on investigation against his instincts and better judgment.

Complications of cross-referrals. The responsibility which the GP has towards his patient is subtly changed when the patient is referred on to hospital, and the responsibility felt by the hospital doctor for the patient may be more indirect as well as affected by

113

the accountability he owes to his superiors, other staff and colleagues of other specialities who may be involved.

Registrar. When I saw the woman the prognosis was not discussed, but she thought she might die. Her main worry was her failing husband. The surgeons sent her to us for treatment of her anaemia and renal failure. Limited efforts were made but the physicians were left feeling uncomfortable. The surgeons implied we were not trying hard enough, and said only a laparotomy would establish whether the mass in her abdomen was malignant or not. We were left to sort this out over a weekend.

GP. The G P probably referred her for perfectly good reasons, but could he have been under pressure to pass her on to the hospital? The surgeons referred her back to the physicians. The buck was passed again. There were various pressures operating in the situation. Did they refer the case to you for assessment or what?

Registrar. I can't remember what the letter actually said. The G P could have sent her to a geriatrician.

QC. What part was played in this case by the relationship between the physicians and surgeons? How much was the discomfort you felt a matter of concern for the patient and how much was it embarrassment before your professional peers?

Physician. It was certainly an embarrassment to have an undiagnosed patient on the ward. It could be taken as a reflection on one's competence.

SW. With whom is the contract? With the patient? or the G P? or the surgeon? Does the situation of cross-referral create a sub-contract between Physician and Surgeon? Is there a dilution of responsibility or a dispersal of responsibility in such situations? Is the physician pressurised more by the surgeon than the needs of the patient?

In theory the doctor's primary responsibility is to the patient, but in practice cross-referrals create complicating extensions to doctor/patient contracts which tend to detract from this primary responsibility. The ancillary responsibilities which the professional acquires in the situation of cross-referral makes him vulnerable to reflections on his professional competence by his peers and staff.

In the case of direct responsibility to the patient, if the individual professional experiences a conflict between his personal feelings and convictions and what is expected of him in his professional role, he has various courses open to him: he can discuss his problem with his peers, with other staff or possibly even with the patient. But in circumstances of cross-referral his professional judgment is at stake and this inhibits him from discussing his problem with others. Although many doctors do consult one another, consultation with others in such circumstances becomes difficult and with the patient virtually impossible. The issue affects his personal self-confidence and his professional credibility. Referring patients on may be a device for avoiding responsibility, but it creates complications. Whether intended or not it creates ambiguities about the nature of the contract with the patient and conflicts of responsibility inevitably arise. The doctor's responsibility *for* his patient may conflict with his responsibility *to* others. Where issues of responsibility and accountability conflict it becomes difficult for different professionals to support one another, because they are put on the defensive. The situation can arise not only in intra-professional relationships between doctors, but in inter-professional relationships between doctors and nurses or between doctors and social workers too.

Registrar. In doing one's job it was almost a question of whether it was a human being who was being hurt or inter-professional and professional relationships which were being damaged.

Psychiatrist. The nurses tend to suggest the doctor should leave the old soul alone. Half say stop, the rest go on! The surgeons drove you.

DN. Nurses often need help when the patient has to face additional suffering, suffering which may appear needless. Doctors proceed along their own lines of scientific investigation which nurses often do not adequately understand, and it isn't explained to them either.

SW. The question is how easy is it to stop and examine what you are doing, to change the direction? There is conflict when we have to put things into reverse gear.

Chaplain. If the GP had shared the Physician's doubts would he have said 'You are dying, we can do tests, but do you want this?'

Registrar. The answer would frequently be: 'Do what you think right, Doctor'.

SW. Pills 4 times a day at home are easy to refuse. But if the patient is in a hospital environment it is difficult for them to refuse treatment.

GP. Part of the difficulty is that the patient can understand pills but cannot understand hospital high technology.

Ward Sister. Patients often confide in the ward sister. What the patient really wants is to be rid of the pain.

QC. Do you pass this on to the Consultant?'

Ward Sister. Yes. I feel I have an obligation to the young nurses and would feel that I have to explain and justify the treatment to them. I have to tell them that the condition may be benign when they suspect otherwise. I have to represent the anxieties of the nurses to the doctors.

Psychiatrist. If 90 per cent of the nurses think it is terrible how strongly do you urge that opinion on the Consultant? The doctor can miss a lot and needs to be kept in touch with the changing circumstances.

Ward Sister. As strongly as possible.

Analysis of conclusions

In discussing decision-making in institutional contexts a number of issues emerged as important: the need to recognise the vulnerability of professionals and the complex emotional demands of terminal care, to distinguish between practical, theoretical and genuine moral dilemmas, to recognise the complexity of relations of responsibility and accountability in professional life, the value of some practical strategies for dealing with moral dilemmas, the need to clarify the relations between personal morality and role-morality.

Emotional demands and the vulnerability of professionals: There is a lack of candidness about the role of feelings in professional practice and an unwillingness to examine these frankly.

The common assumption (pace Talcott Parsons) that the professional is supposed to maintain an attitude of detachment ('affective neutrality') towards patients/clients was seriously questioned. While useful in certain circumstances, particularly in emergencies and acute medicine, it was inappropriate to longer-term caring relationships (e.g. in psychiatry, in social work, in nursing long-stay patients and in terminal care). In cases of death and bereavement it is not necessarily 'unprofessional' or a 'sign of inadequate professionalisation' for the doctor, nurse, minister or social worker to show emotion. It would be unnatural for them to hide their feelings in a situation which demanded a response of simple humanity rather than clinical detachment.

To communicate with patients as persons, the professional should admit to himself the nature of his feelings about the patient/client. Professionals do in fact find some individuals 'attractive', others 'repulsive', some 'difficult' others 'compliant', some 'rewarding to work with', others not. This needs to be admitted if they are not to deceive themselves about the motives of self-interest and desire for fulfilment which play a part in professional commitment to service and determine whether the professional finds his job rewarding or not. Professional detachment should never be achieved at the price of bad faith. Professional confidence, a capacity to empathise and show compassion even towards the unattractive and difficult patient are built more easily on honesty about feelings. Learning when it is appropriate to show emotion, and when it should be avoided if possible, requires both experience and honesty in the recognition of the feelings present in particular professional/client relationships.

The professional needs to recognise his own feelings and anxieties about death, how they affect his professional performance, and how fear of the emotional and psychological distress associated with death and bereavement may cause him to withdraw from those who need his support. The 'bereavement of the professional' may be a very real experience in some circumstances too —not only when the patient is well known to the professional, but when death makes the professional painfully aware of his own impotence or ignorance of how to cope with a particular crisis. It is important that there should be better preparation of professionals to face the ordeal of a death where they are professionally involved —by appropriate 'de-briefing' and the provision of better intra-professional support.

The privilege of intimacy which the professional shares with the patient/client can create difficulties too—where the professional is called on to advise in a non-professional role, e.g. in giving moral advice or spiritual counsel. The physical intimacy of medical and nursing contacts with patients, the privileged access which health-care professionals enjoy when invited into people's homes, the confidentiality of the relationship in the consulting professions (including s w's and Ministers), all create responsibilities which extend beyond the strictly defined professional role. The boundaries of the Curing, Caring and Counselling roles are never precise and tend to become blurred as management changes from curative to terminal care. The confidence of the dying patient in a particular professional and dependence on him may mean in practice that he is expected to perform all three roles at once. Where the beliefs or value-system of professional or patient differ it may be particularly difficult for the professional—who has to choose between dissembling, passing the responsibility to someone else, or being frank and sincere. Again clear recognition of the feelings involved is a necessary base for sound decisions.

The professional, and especially the doctor, is trained to be a self-reliant individual. He is in effect a trained soloist accustomed to make decisions and to carry responsibility on his own. Consequently he may experience difficulty in admitting to himself the limits of his power and competence, or admitting that he cannot cope with his responsibilities and needs support. Admission of these things to a colleague is felt to amount almost to an admission of failure. There is an associated risk therefore that society will expect too much of the doctor and other professionals—encouraging them to 'pass the buck' when they cannot cope. The doctor, for example, not only has to decide on treatment, but has to decide when a professional response is inappropriate—when further investigations and treatment are unnecessary. Such decisions are not easily shared and guilt and anxiety may be associated with specific decisions for years afterward ('perhaps we should have tried harder . . .').

Theoretical, Practical and Moral Dilemmas. There is a need to distinguish between different kinds of dilemmas—theoretical, practical and moral—because these present different kinds of problems and require different kinds of strategies to resolve them.

In the case of a theoretical dilemma where alternative explanations of the same phenomena are possible, the anxiety centres on right knowledge or understanding. If the explanation of the aetiology of a disease is uncertain and rival theories exist, only further research and argument about the adequacy of different explanations can possibly decide the issue. The clinician may be bothered by the uncertainty that exists in terms of being able to give convincing explanations of his diagnoses, but theoretical disagreements in medicine need not affect his clinical practice, in the sense of his ability to diagnose and treat in terms of whichever explanation appeals to him (e.g. in disagreements about the causes of hypertension or schizophrenia).

In the case of practical dilemmas, where alternative and equally sensible courses of action seem possible (as in choosing between surgery or further barium studies in the case in question) the anxiety centres on the need to get something done. As long as the problem is seen simply as a practical and technical one the issue can be decided only by the quest for further information and by technical investigation. Where the evidence is ambiguous and alternative diagnoses are possible the urgent need is for more evidence which may hopefully decide the issue and yield a clear diagnosis in terms of which decisions can be made about further treatment. The logic of clinical practice commits the doctor faced with a practical dilemma to continue investigation in the hope of eliminating uncertainty. However, certainty is rarely possible and other human and moral considerations tend to come into play, inhibiting his quest for scientific truth and reassuring certainty.

Because the practice of medicine involves people and people base their choices on values of various kinds, decisions in clinical practice cannot avoid moral issues. Choices may have to be made between different sets of values. It is not always appreciated by the public that a certain amount of what doctors decide and advise necessarily involves both factual- and value-judgments.

In a situation in which there is a genuine moral dilemma the issue cannot be decided simply by appeal to rules, for in the nature of the case there are different sets of rules and these are in conflict with one another. Similarly, there can be no universal practical rule for dealing with moral dilemmas for either there would be no dilemma or the situation demands a decision, a moral choice which involves, by definition, the courage to cut out certain alternatives and possibilities.

Confronted with moral dilemmas, professionals often become victims of the 'Something must be done' syndrome, instead of facing up to the fact that a value-judgment is required. The professional attempts to resolve the moral dilemma by defining it as a 'problem', that is as something to which his own knowledge and expertise is applicable. The attempt is made to translate the moral dilemma into a practical dilemma, that is, as something which the individual can manage in the accustomed professional manner, and where responsibility is limited to the efficient performance of a pre-scribed function. This strategy for avoiding moral responsibility by falling back on professional efficiency was seen as a means of dodging the issue of moral choice involved. Like falling back on authority ('If only there were a senior consultant here to decide') such strategies were seen as attempts to abrogate responsibility or to 'pass the buck'.

Responsibility and accountability in institutional contexts. In practice the moral autonomy of the individual doctor or nurse, social worker or minister may be severely limited. The nearer the situation is to a direct one-to-one doctor/patient or professional/client relationship, the easier it is for the individual to exercise moral autonomy (i.e. to act as a self-regulating, self-legislating agent). Once the individual professional becomes involved in the health-care team with other professionals, the exercise of responsibility becomes more complicated. The doctor may retain responsibility for the decisions of the health-care team, in the sense of being the one who is legally accountable, but he can no longer act independently or with complete autonomy. In principle he is committed to responsible consultation and some of his functions may have to be delegated, the special knowledge and expertise of other professionals has to be recognised. In hospital, the institutional setting, the division of work between various departments and specialities, and the hierarchical system of authority further limits the individual's professional and moral autonomy, making it more difficult to find creative solutions to moral dilemmas in particular cases.

For the GP or SW confronted with the individual patient/client it may be possible to resolve a moral dilemma *ad hoc*—by a pragmatic approach based on trial and error. In the context of team co-operation the resolution of dilemmas becomes more difficult. Not only do more people have to be consulted, but specific solutions worked out in particular cases would tend to become precedents. In institutional settings these difficulties would be even greater, requiring a greater degree of moral discrimination and maturity to cope with them.

The wider consultation required in the health-care team creates anxiety and frustration unless someone is prepared to accept responsibility for making a decision. This means that the pressures on the doctor may be much greater than in the consulting room—for he has not only to respond to pressures from the patient and family, but also from nurses, social workers and other medical colleagues. In such a situation a dilemma shared may become a dilemma multiplied. The unwillingness of one individual to take a responsible decision on his own may simply mean that many more people become involved in his problem making it more difficult rather than easier to find a solution. The dispersal of responsibility in a situation where there is no clear definition of the locus of authority, can make it much worse. The sharing of responsibility can only be a constructive means of dealing with practical problems if there is common agreement as to who should exercise authority in a particular situation and common willingness to stand by that individual when he decides.

The changing pattern in health-care, with an increasing tendency to abolish hierarchical authority has the benefit in theory of giving the individual clinician more autonomy, but given the team context in which he operates it also means that he carries more responsibility in a situation where his authority is more ambiguous. Where the doctor remains legally accountable he may wish to assert his authority without adequate consultation with other members of the team. This may cause friction and misunderstanding and unwillingness of members to share responsibility and give support to the doctor. The clear recognition of the circumstances when the authority lies with the doctor and when for example it might shift to the social worker, is necessary if the relative responsibility and authority of each is to be recognised and respected. Too much stress on the desirability of professional autonomy fails to do justice to the reality of inter-professional dependence (e.g. of the dependence of nurses on doctors, doctors on social workers and vice-versa). It also fails to do justice to the realities of peer-group answerability among colleagues (between different doctors, between nurses, between social workers and between chaplains). The dependence too of junior doctors on senior doctors, junior nurses on their seniors, means that in practice the exercise of responsibility takes place under the critical gaze of others who may or are entitled to criticise his actions. The individual may find it more difficult to face the anticipated criticism of his professional peers or superiors, who serve as arbiters of his actions, than to face the responsibility of a difficult choice in relation to a dependent patient/client.

Practical strategies for dealing with moral dilemmas. Nevertheless it was recognised that there are various practical strategies for dealing with moral dilemmas:

First, the individual must admit to himself the nature of the problem and seek to identify what the conflicting values in the situation are. 'Some choices are inevitably difficult, but at least we can ensure that we know what we are doing and can offer a reasonable justification for our action.'

Second, the individual can seek to assess the degree of his own personal responsibility in the situation—so that in his anxiety he does not either exaggerate it or abrogate responsibility for what he should do. 'If only we could all frankly say: "A bit of it's mine". "I'm not sure how much, but I'm prepared to shoulder my share of responsibility." '

Third, the individual can share with his peers and colleagues possible ways of dealing with the problem: 'When I meet dilemmas I collect views, weigh up the fors and againsts. It makes me feel better. Sometimes the shape of the problem changes in the process and it becomes more manageable.'

Fourth, it may be possible for the individual to look objectively at the balance of probabilities, to make a factual assessment, and then attempt to de-sensitise himself to the problem by discussing it with someone who is not emotionally involved.

Finally, if the problem remains intractable the only alternatives are either to procrastinate or act in the spirit of trial and error—attempting with confidence to choose the lesser of two evils or the best course available.

If there is a genuine moral dilemma, in principle, there is no rule which can decide how you should act. You either avoid making a decision or in fear and trembling pioneer a new initiative. The resolution of moral dilemmas in practice requires moral courage and a willingness of the individual or team to attempt a new solution, a new approach in the light of the particular situation. This means choosing neither horn of the dilemma, but attempting to

121

transcend both alternatives by a creative response to the needs of the particular situation—recognising that it cannot serve as a precedent but only as a solution appropriate to this particular case. Such solutions are not generalisable and no universal rules are deducible from particular courageous initiatives, but each responsible attempt to deal with such dilemmas makes it easier for others to follow and work out similar solutions for themselves.

Personal morality and role-morality. The predicament of people in large institutions is that they are often required to accept responsibility without commensurate power. It is necessary for the efficient functioning of institutions that certain individuals are answerable for what goes on, but in practice responsibility may actually be shared by many others. (See Emmet 1966, p 201)

> In any formal institution there must be some people who, in virtue of their office, are responsible in the sense of answerable for decisions, policies and their outcome. This need not mean that they had a major share in making the decision (they may even have their own reservations about it, or not have been able to prevent what happened). They have, however, to be prepared to take public responsibility without disclosing their private reservations or giving away confidential matter on how the decision was taken (for some things must be discussed confidentially), and particularly they must be prepared to 'carry the can' if things go wrong. This is a feature of the nature of constitutional responsibility in institutional life. . . .

Dilemmas of personal and professional responsibility are thus experienced by the individual as he moves out of the simple face-to-face situation into social and institutional contexts where he has to make decisions which involve numerous people in different ways— either as those who suffer the direct consequences of his actions or those who are indirectly affected by his action or those who are subject to his authority, or those to whom he is answerable. The resolution of dilemmas involving conflicts between the different values governing these different roles will be partly a matter of individual moral courage and initiative, it will be partly a function of growth in experience and sophistication in living through the complex morality of institutions in a personally authentic way.

SUGGESTED READING FOR CHAPTER SEVEN

The studies listed in the Bibliography under British Medical Association (1974), Campbell (1972), Central Council (1976), Downie (1971), Eadie (1975), Emmet (1966), Friedson (1975), McFarlane (1976), McGilloway (1976), Mitchell (1976), Parsons (1951), Thompson (1976).

EIGHT

Conflicts of Values in Inter-Professional Decision-Making

THIS CHAPTER examines the problems of decision-making in terminal care of an acute accident case by a team of specialists. The effect of different professional values in determining attitudes and complicating the task of reaching agreement on the ward is considered, and the function of institutional and legal factors examined.

The basic values of Medicine, Nursing, Social Work and the Ministry are examined briefly on the basis of existing Codes of Ethics and official Declaration in the first three, and common elements in the values of the caring professions noted, together with their common origins in the religious and moral traditions of our culture.

The case presented concerns a young patient in a neuro-surgery department who has been fatally injured. The parents rather surprisingly request that no attempt should be made to save the boy's life. The consultant and ward staff are disturbed by this. A night nurse refuses to administer the prescribed pain-relieving injection. The patient recovers consciousness in a state of anxiety and distress, further upsetting the staff. This causes conflict between the staff and the attempt by the consultant to call a case-conference to achieve consensus and co-operation between the staff is only partially successful.

The issues discussed cover the night-nurse's 'right' to conscientious objection to what she regards as euthanasia, different models for inter-professional co-operation, the dependence of different professionals on one another. In analysing these issues the following questions were considered: the problems of inter-professional teams, the value and significance of case-conferences, and finally the nature of values themselves and their relation to practice.

The Medical Profession
Although the Hippocratic Oath and the International Code of

123

Medical Ethics set out in different ways the values of the medical profession, the Ethical Code of the Commonwealth Medical Association (1974) does so in a particularly clear and succinct way: 1. The doctor's primary loyalty is to his patient. 2. His vocation and skill shall be devoted to the amelioration of symptoms, the cure of illness, and the promotion of health. 3. He shall respect human life and studiously avoid doing it injury. 4. He shall share all the knowledge he may have gained with his colleagues without reserve. 5. He shall respect the confidence of his patient as he would his own. 6. He shall by precept and example maintain the dignity and ideals of the profession, and permit no bias based on race, creed or socio-economic factors to affect his professional practice.

While there may be consensus that these values characterise medical practice in general, how they will be interpreted in practice may vary from one context to another. It is a common sociological observation that values are functionally related to different work settings and therefore it follows that the interpretation of the doctor's ethical code will vary according to whether he is functioning mainly as a consulting clinician, as a caring person, as a research scientist, or as a medical administrator.

In discussing 'the clinical mentality' in his book *Profession of Medicine* (1970) Eliot Friedson argues that the values of the individual clinician are related to the peculiar nature of the context in which he has to exercise medical responsibility—where he has to take risks in the course of medical intervention. Consequently the values which characterise his work are pragmatism, individualism and a sense of vulnerability or uncertainty. Both his medical and moral judgments tend to be of a trial-and-error nature, based on what he knows to work on the basis of knowledge and past experience. His orientation is towards the needs of the individual patient rather than the common good, and he is inclined to emphasise the need for individual choice based on first-hand experience because of the uncertain state of medical knowledge and the deficiencies of available techniques.

The particularism and moral subjectivity characteristic of the clinical man's work does not mean that he is not rational. . . . The difference between clinical rationality and scientific rationality is that clinical rationality is not a tool for the exploration or discovery of general principles, as is the scientific method, but only a tool for sorting the interconnections of perceived and hypothesised facts.

While the demands of the caring role will also lead to an emphasis on an individual and case-based approach to clinical and moral problems, the demands of medical research and health-care plan-

124

ning and administration will lead to a more universalistic emphasis on the common good, on the need for general rules and for more formal definition of professional roles and an ethic of duty.

The Nursing Profession

The same conflicts are common to the other professions. They are perhaps particularly acute in nursing—where the individual nurse may be torn between her duty to one specific patient and her duties to other patients on the ward or in the hospital. The disagreements about the value of 'task-centred' or 'patient-centred' approaches to nursing care hinge on different interpretations of nursing values.

The International Council of Nurses' Code for Nurses emphasises the following values as fundamental to nursing: 'The fundamental responsibility of the nurse is fourfold: to promote health, to prevent illness, to restore health and to alleviate suffering. The need for nursing is universal. Inherent in nursing is respect for life, dignity and rights of man. It is unrestricted by considerations of nationality, race, creed, colour, sex, politics or social status. Nurses render health services to the individual, the family and the community and coordinate their services with those of related groups. The nurse's primary responsibility is to those people who require nursing care. The nurse, in providing care, promotes an environment in which the values, customs and spiritual beliefs of the individual are respected. The nurse holds in confidence personal information and uses judgment in sharing this information.

In addition to these values which relate to the professional/client relationship the ICN Code and the Royal College of Nursing Code both emphasise the responsibilities of nurses to maintain high standards of training, to promote public health, and to act as an advocate in the patient's cause, to protect their autonomy and to protect them from neglect or abuse. However, the nurse is also 'under an obligation to carry out the physician's orders intelligently and loyally and to refuse to participate in unethical procedures'. This means that there may well be conflicts of conscience for the individual nurse when her duty to carry out orders conflicts either with her assessment of the patient's needs and condition, or where it conflicts with her own personal moral convictions. The nurse, unlike the doctor, can be involved in a 'double bind' situation —of a conflict of duties based on different professional values, and personal conflict between professional and personal moral duties. (Conflicts over appropriate levels of pain relief, or the termination of life-support may have this character for nurses.)

The Social Work Profession

As a fairly new profession Social Workers have devoted a considerable amount of attention to the clarification of the value-bases of Social Work. The British Association of Social Workers recently convened a special multi-disciplinary working party to examine the subject and its publication, *Values in Social Work* represents an impressive attempt to consider the relations of Social Workers not only to clients and the public, but to other professionals.

The BASW *Code of Ethics for Social Work* (1975) expresses the fundamental values of social work in the following terms: Basic to the profession of social work is the recognition of the value and dignity of every human being irrespective of origin, status, sex, age, belief or contribution to society. The profession accepts responsibility to encourage and facilitate the self-realisation of the individual person with due regard for the interests of others.

Like other professional codes the sw code emphasises the importance of confidentiality while recognising the conflicting interests that may qualify it as an ultimate value. However, the chief values emphasised are the acceptance of people whatever their estate, to enhance their power of self-determination and to act as an advocate in the cause of the weak and helpless. 'These aims mean assisting people to define and anticipate problems vis-à-vis their social environment; to help people recognise and develop their own coping and problem-solving capacities; to link people with others and systems which can provide them with the resources and services they require; to encourage in these systems a sensitive, humane and effective practice in response to the needs of their consumers; to contribute to the instigation, maintenance and development of responsible and constructive social policy; to carry out the responsibilities which society has accepted in respect of those children for whom adequate care is not being provided; and for those adults who are unable to care for themselves; to act on behalf of society, as agents of social control, in accordance with these values, rather than to abdicate this role to other persons or organisations whose functioning is not caring based; and, finally to offer practical material assistance so far as this is consistent with upholding the autonomy and dignity of the client.' (Musselburgh Social Work Department Memo, 1976.)

The Ministry

The status of the ministry as a Consulting, Scholarly or Caring profession is ambiguous. In practice it has elements of all three.

Historically the priesthood or ministry has set the standards for the other caring professions—particularly since medical and nursing, and indirectly social work, functions have been historically linked to the functions of religious orders. The values of altruistic service, non-discrimination, client advocacy, confidentiality, reverence for life and defence of the dignity of the individual all have a respectable theological heritage—whatever abuses they have been subject to in the history of religion. However, the specific values of the ministry, apart from the transcendent theological functions of prophetic criticism, moral guidance and priestly intercession, tend to focus in practice on the function of the minister as the caring individual par excellence.

An idealised self-image (cf. K. Horney), based on ideals of being loving and lovable, is the springboard for 'the helping personality'. The clergyman sees himself as being essentially loving and is motivated by the wish to be a helpful, loving, considerate, concerned, compassionate and affectionate person. This is the ideal which he strives to attain. (Eadie, H.A., 1975, p. 2.)

The minister or chaplain has the role of trying to be an exemplary caring person. This is both the blessing and the curse of his position. He represents in some sense the transcendent ideals of self-less service and is doubly vulnerable to criticism in his attempt to exercise his caring and counselling functions. He has also to simultaneously represent the demands of an ethic of love which places an infinite value on each individual in his unique situation, and the universal and institutionalised values of a culture which is nominally religious. In the hospital, he may be revered as the friend and confidant of patients and professionals alike or resented as an implied judge of the moral and spiritual standards of those around.

Case presentation

Transaction: spinal cord. Ischaemic damage—progressive and permanent. Presented by a ward sister.

'David'

David, aged 13 years, was the only child of middle-aged parents. He was attending a public school as a 'day boy'. Playing a 'banned' game—a special form of leap-frog—another boy landed right on his neck.

Day 1. On admission to paediatric neurosurgical unit, already very clear evidence of spinal cord damage. Loss of movement and sensation in lower limbs up as far as lower abdomen. A handsome

127

boy, large and obviously physically very fit, who was fully conscious and very anxious.

Over the next few hours his condition deteriorated, the level of loss of function rose. A tracheostomy was performed under local anaesthetic, to enable a respirator to be used. David, responding to sedation and constant reassurance from the medical and nursing staff, coped extraordinarily well with this unpleasant procedure.

The consultant, who was pessimistic about the possibility of recovery of the cord from the damage, had a long session with David's parents. David was kept fairly heavily sedated and given 'Constant Care' nursing.

Day 2. David suffered total loss of all sensation and function of the upper limbs. The parents visited and asked if there was any hope of recovery. They were told as gently as possible by the consultant that he believed there was no hope. He discussed David's possible future as a quadriplegic. The ward sister was also present. The parents saw David and went out for lunch.

They returned after several hours, and asked to speak to the consultant. They requested that no further efforts should be made to prolong David's life and asked that he should not be allowed to suffer. The consultant was surprised and disturbed by their response and suggested a second opinion. The parents did not feel this was necessary but the consultant insisted. The second opinion confirmed the same diagnosis and prognosis.

A 'case conference' was convened by the consultant, involving the ward sister, staff nurse, registrar and the anaesthetist who operated the respirator. A decision was eventually reached to discontinue antibiotics, to provide suction to the tracheostomy only if the patient was distressed, and to increase sedation.

Day 3. David was found wide awake, alert and very anxious. The night nurse had withheld 2 doses of sedation because he was asleep (in spite of formal instruction that 'sedation to be given 4 hourly'). She said it was against her religion to give drugs unnecessarily. David asked to see the ward sister as soon as she appeared on duty. He asked her if he was dying. This she denied vehemently and spent some time with him talking to him.

The parents visited later in the day and when he was asleep they came in to say goodbye. They never returned. David slept most of the day and sedation was given regularly. He had ice-cream and 'sherry with lemonade' to drink when he was awake, as this was his favourite tipple.

That night there was a different night nurse on duty, because

128

the consultant had intervened and had the other removed.

Day 4. No sedation needed. David died at approximately 1 p.m.

Comment by GP. Some reflections on the characters in the drama:
The Consultant: He is the key figure in this drama. The staff rely on
his experience, training and confidence. In the crisis he behaves
paradoxically—first in a very capable way and then is disturbed
by the unexpected reaction of the parents and their request to
terminate treatment. His lack of confidence upsets the team,
upsets the harmony of the ward. What was it about the parents'
reaction that upset him? Was it that they were so completely
willing to accept his verdict? Was it because he was aware of the
dependence of the nurses on him, of how his uncertainty upset
them? The question is to whom do doctors turn for help and
support in a crisis—seeking or advising a second opinion is only
part of the solution? *The Parents*: Their reaction upset the whole
medical team, doctors and nurses. Why? The parents did not
stay with the child. Why? Was it really their decision or were
they influenced by hospital policy? Were they already anticipating bereavement and thus withdrawing from a reality too painful to face? Was it not possible for them to have been seen by a
social worker or chaplain? Perhaps it all happened so quickly
that nothing could really be done for them. *The Ward Sister*:
Nurses were obviously affected by the general tension. The night
nurse's religious convictions have to be respected. She should
perhaps have explained her difficulty to the ward sister, but to
whom could she turn for support in a moral crisis when she disagreed with the rest of the staff? The ward sister's reaction on
finding the boy awake and distressed is understandable—she
was the one in whom the boy had chosen to confide. From whom
could she seek support? The consultant's severe reaction to the
disobedience of the night nurse could only aggravate the tension
between the staff. *The Case-conference.* The key questions raised
by the case-conference relate to: i) The issue of inter-professional dependency and conflict and the question of who supports
whom; ii) The issue of whether the case-conference was a means
of sharing responsibility, or avoiding it, and whether it was an
effective way of reaching a consensus decision or an indirect way
by which the consultant sought reinforcement of his own
decision; iii) Finally there is the question of whether the parents
should have been involved?

Comment by SW. Does the fact that the parents took the initiative mean that they pre-empted the initiative and authority of the
consultant, taking part of his role away and so leaving him feel-

ing undermined? It seems to be implied in this instance that the fact that the consultant sought a second opinion reflects on his competence and management of the case. Is it necessary to dress up the consultant's need for support as a quest for more scientific information? Why could this need not have been shared with the group? Is this in part the source of the stress?

Perhaps the night nurse was fortunate to have a religion—to have external reasons for not giving sedation to the sleeping boy. She had a let-out for not doing what she (and probably other nurses without such an excuse) would not have wanted to do. It was her way of dressing up her right to challenge authority on a matter of feeling and conscience.

Perhaps the child was fortunate to be a child—to have had his whims pampered. Could this not be extended to adults in such circumstances? Can't the rules be bent more often in caring for the dying? How often are the interests of the dying submerged in the need to maintain hospital discipline or routine?

The direct challenge from the child to the ward sister: 'Am I going to die?' must have been particularly stressful, as there was no time or opportunity in this case for the issue to be gone through and talked over with the child. The issue of telling children would always be more problematic as they would not be likely to understand or just be frightened—especially when it is realised that there can be no second opportunity. This would have left the ward sister particularly vulnerable and in need of support.

Illustrative discussion

Discussions began with consideration of the responsibilities of the nurse, and whether she had a right to challenge the authority of the consultant or ward sister. There was considerable sympathy evoked for the night nurse, with one doctor saying that he would expect her to show initiative and discretion in the interpretation of his instructions. Nurses in the group insisted that she had acted illegally and that as a junior nurse she had no choice but to act in terms of the letter of her written instructions or hand over to someone else.

Sister. Had the night nurse the right on religious grounds to refuse to give the sedation? Did that give her the right to decide what was in the best interests of the child?

Chaplain. She was a devoutly religious girl and had strong views about euthanasia. She was clearly afraid that there was something on the go and didn't want to be responsible.

Nurse-tutor. The question is whether she understood her legal

130

obligations. She could refuse to give it herself but she ought to have consulted with other nursing staff.

Physician A. She was faced with the simple problem: Do I wake the patient?

Nurse-tutor. If the drugs are written up, they must be given.

Physician B. She could have consulted with other staff or asked the doctor.

Sister. Sharing is an ideal, it doesn't happen often enough in practice.

Chaplain. Nurses are understandably afraid to give what might be the last injection—and it is difficult to be the odd man out on the team. She has my sympathy.

GP. All hell was let loose the following day—the night nurse was removed.

Nurse-tutor. It still would happen today.

GP. The instructions cannot be always sufficiently clear, nor is it always possible to bring in the nurses, they must use some discretion.

Nurse-tutor. The point about team-work is important, but there can be no argument about the drugs. The nurse's legal responsibility is to fulfil her instructions.

Physician A. No damage resulted from the failure to sedate the boy—except that it provoked an emotional crisis for the ward sister.

SW. Surely this is an issue of communication and not a mere legal issue? The question is one of sharing knowledge and responsibility. Did she know and understand why the drugs were necessary? Could she be expected to carry the responsibility without being adequately informed? Her religious beliefs simply provided the ground for refusing to accept responsibility for a decision in which she had no real part.

GP. The ward sister was thrown off balance by finding the boy awake and was challenged by his agitated question whether he was dying. She implied: 'If he had been sedated, he wouldn't have asked me.'

Physician A. She was grabbed by that patient. (Dying patients do look round for the right person to speak to.)

SW. Yes. And was not the night nurse the unfortunate scapegoat for the ward sister's distress and the consultant's anxiety?

Physician B. I would say unquestionably no. She did not consult the senior nurses before taking a very important decision. It was nothing to do with anybody's distress and anxiety.

Nurse-tutor. But there is often real friction between doctors and nurses about drugs. There is a need for more real respect for each other's expertise but also about each other's respective legal responsibilities. Nurses often have to instruct residents on the legalities of drug administration.

Psychiatrist. What people are anxious about in such circumstances are questions like 'What would I say in court?' or 'What would the papers say?'

Sister. I can take some risks with the law because I have indemnity insurance, but student nurses are obliged to stick to the letter of the law. Sisters can take some independent responsibility.

GP. Doctors do delegate responsibility to nurses and expect them to use their initiative.

Physician B. Or is this just 'passing the buck'? The nurses here have not indicated that they are willing to take responsibility for decisions. On the contrary they have taken refuge in discussion of their legal responsibilities.

The night nurse's dilemma was not simply a matter of conscience but another example of how the exercise of moral responsibility is complicated by the institutional setting within which it has to be exercised. In established institutions such as hospitals, with their traditional hierarchical structure, authority is delegated and exercised within a framework of rules and legal requirements. It cannot be exercised on the basis of informal understanding, unless new structures and new rules are created to give definition to the roles and responsibilities of the co-operative team.

Different models for inter-professional co-operation. Two models were considered: first what was called 'the Social Work model', and second, 'the traditional hospital model'. The characteristics of the first were given as: the emphasis on open consultation and co-operation of the professionals as a team, the recognition of the need for a more flexible approach to confidentiality on the team with more direct consultation with clients about the limits of confidentiality, and more explicit negotiation of professional/client contracts. The hospital model was seen as more legalistic and authoritarian, based on an explicit hierarchy among nursing and medical staff with the delegation of responsibility from above according to explicit rules and established procedures. In modern health-care and hospital medicine there tends to be tension between the two models. In areas of medicine where social problems are of central importance—e.g. in psychiatry and geriatric medicine, in ante-natal and post-natal obstetrics, and paediatric medicine and in terminal care—the 'Social Work' team model seems to have more relevance and direct application. In acute medicine of all kinds, in situations demanding decisive action, efficiency and speed, the hierarchical model appears to be better suited to the circumstances ('Rules and discipline, and clearly defined lines of authority are necessary in situations of stress and emergency').

The banning of the night nurse from the ward was as much a response to the stressful situation and the need to find a scapegoat, as a matter of discipline and sticking to the rules. In the conflict which arose over the disobedience of the night nurse 'the legal issue was less important than the issue of the appropriate framework of communication'. The need for more open consultation between the nurses and between the nursing staff and the medical staff was only partly met by the case-conference, there remained a conflict between the hierarchical order of actual relationships and the attempted form of team consultation. The advantages of open consultation on the team with the corresponding confidence in shared responsibility, is offset by the disadvantages that it is very time-consuming and may lead to delay and indecision unless there is clear leadership of the team. The advantages of the more authoritarian model— that it is supposedly more efficient and allows the doctor opportunity to exercise his leadership of the clinical team—are offset by the fact that this system does not allow for the use of initiative and full responsibility by the other and more numerous members of the health-care team.

This led to consideration of the changing role of the nurse, particularly in the context of terminal care. It was recognised that with increased training and expertise the balance of responsibility in decision-making is changing and that in the ward case-conference or in the PMCT the views of the nursing staff are increasingly important and sometimes decisive. In discussion the nurses vigorously defended the view that the nurse has a dual role—the medically delegated role ('Handmaiden') and an independent role based on her specialised skills. The doctors lamented the passing of the traditional nurse-handmaiden while maintaining that nurses should be treated as equals and expected on the one hand 'to use their discretion', but on the other hand insisted that 'the doctor is the natural leader of the team—because of the wider spectrum of his knowledge'. However, it was agreed that in certain circumstances the nurse's share of responsibility for a particular decision (e.g. in determining the level of pain control) might be greater than the doctor's, and that conflicts arise when doctors fail to recognise this. The dynamics of sharing responsibility in decision-making are not to be confused with the legal responsibility of the doctor to the patient, as the contracting party. It is a question of the proper demarcation of roles.

While the demands of team-medicine make it necessary for wide

133

consultation to take place and while in different situations the nurse or some other member of the team may have to take responsible decisions, the institutional and legal responsibilities of the doctor mean that he has to 'carry the can' even if he disagrees with the decision which has been taken.

The dependence of different professionals on one another. An important factor in inter-professional co-operation, particularly in stressful situations,was seen to be the mutual dependence of different professionals for support of both a practical and emotional kind.

1st Physician. There is no question of 'dressing up the consultant's need for support', as the s w suggests. He wanted reconsideration of the hard facts of what was an extremely important case, where there could be no second chance.

2nd Physician. However, the fact that the consultant in this case wavered caused uncertainty and even distress to the nurses and other staff who depended on him.

Nurse. But it was obvious that the consultant depended too on the support of the nursing staff to bolster his confidence that he had made the right decisions.

SW. Why should we regard it as so frightfully important that the doctor or the ward sister should act independently? Why should it matter that they were dependent on one another for support? Surely it is perfectly reasonable that there should be a strong element of dependency in inter-professional relationships as in ordinary human relations? It would be alarming if nurses or social workers in trying to establish their own legitimate role were to isolate themselves from their fellow professionals. We mustn't ascribe a negative quality to dependency. It is the independent exercise of authority that we should perhaps question.

1st Physician. This is true but the patient should see only one end opinion and action, not conflicting opinions and actions.

GP. Given the dual roles of the modern nurse—as 'handmaiden' and as independent contractor with special skills of her own—is she any longer so dependent on the doctor?

Nurse. With changes in the nurse's 'handmaiden' role she is less dependent on the doctor. Nurses are more able to give one another support.

1st Physician. Is this dependency on others emotional? It is more a dependency on others for information and expertise. I depend on my nurses for hard information about patients when I am not there.

Nurse. The fact that you call them 'my nurses' shows that the dependence is not just formal but also personal.

134

Both over-rigid hierarchical arrangements and the self-conscious assertion of independence by individual professional groups (e.g. by doctors, nurses or social workers) denies the essential elements of authority and dependency in all human and institutional relationships. The authority of the doctor is not incompatible with his dependence on nursing and social work staff for different kinds of information, assistance and support. Likewise the authority of the ward-sister or district nurse may at times bring her into opposition with the doctor but she needs his co-operation and support as much as her junior nurses need both her authority and support. Thus the case-conference in the case under discussion represented both an attempt to reach a consensus decision and an attempt to resolve inter-professional anxiety and conflict.

It was agreed that the source of the uncertainty and conflict was not the absence of a decision or the fact that the wrong decision was taken—'Parents and consultants were both right. There was no reversible lesion. The trauma was the boy's. Decisions were made. Both were proved right.' The sense of disquiet left after the boy's death could be attributed to the unsatisfactory relationship of the medical and nursing staff to the parents on the one hand, and to the fact that the boy was found alert and anxious when it was hoped that he would be unconscious. The chief source of the difficulty was the fact that 'somewhere the decision was disallowed, interpreted differently'. The consultant acted in such a way as to suggest that he felt his decision-making initiative and authority had been undermined by the parents. The consultant and other staff felt that their group decision-making authority (including the will of the parents) had been challenged by the defiant action of the night nurse. The speed of events and lack of time for discussion or adjustment heightened the tension. It was felt that the conflict of authority which arose between consultant and parents was apparent rather than real and that the consultant's anxiety arose with the responsibility of being the last arbiter. 'Most consultants are not unwilling to consult others if uncertain what to do. You are glad to share it, pleased to be proved wrong.'

Analysis of conclusions

Several issues emerged out of discussion: the problems of inter-professional team co-operation, the value and significance of the inter-professional case-conference, and the question of the nature of values themselves.

The problems of inter-professional teams. The absence of clear definitions of professional roles, in situations demanding inter-professional co-operation, and accompanying uncertainty about the scope and limits of professional responsibility, was seen as a prime cause of misunderstanding. Because professionals tend to be soloists—accustomed to exercise their own judgment, act independently and accept responsibility for their actions—they are not particularly suited by training or experience to co-operate in teams. If this situation is to be changed a number of things have to be recognised: i) the inadequacy of present training for the experience of inter-professional team work, ii) the inadequacy of present mechanisms for inter-professional consultation over common problems, iii) the inadequacy of inter- and intra-professional support systems for professionals operating in situations of stress such as terminal care.

The separate training of Doctors, Nurses, Social Workers, Ministers and other health-care professionals is necessary in specialised areas, but it is appropriate that they should have some training in common if they are to work together, and, it was argued, common training would encourage each professional group to understand and respect the other's functions better. Common training and shared experience would also help trainees to develop appropriate mechanisms for inter-professional consultation, make them aware of the different stresses to which each kind of professional is subject, and encourage the formation of intra-professional and inter-professional support groups.

Second, it was recognised that the effectiveness of professional services, especially in health-care, depends to some extent on 'the placebo effect', i.e. the efficacy of patient/client trust in the authority of the professional. Delegation and dispersal of responsibility on the health-care team makes individual professionals uneasy about their authority in relation to their patient/client. The charisma of the professional is partly a function of his particular knowledge and skills, partly of his personal authority, partly of his individual personality. These things tend to have less importance in the more egalitarian atmosphere of the health-care team, and individual professionals felt there was some loss of prestige and influence with patients/clients in these circumstances and risk that professional responsibility in therapeutic relationships would not be taken so seriously. Doctors in particular felt that there was a clash between the autonomy required for the exercise of proper clinical judgment, and the inter-dependence required in the situation of shared team responsibility.

The demands of acute therapeutic medicine for efficiency and decisiveness, favour a situation in which authority is exercised in an hierarchical order, with final authority being vested in the doctor. The demands of caring, supportive and counselling roles, as in long-stay or terminal care favour more active involvement of nursing, social work, counselling and other rehabilitative health-care staff and hence of a more democratic and shared system of authority. The conflict between these two models was seen to be particularly relevant to terminal care where the switch from an aggressive therapeutic regime to terminal care may not involve corresponding changes in the organisation of inter-professional relationships. When the whole process of terminal management from the pre-death to dying phase is controlled in the same environment by the Primary Medical Care Team, or Hospital Staff, where each group is accustomed to functioning in a democratic or hierarchical order, there is not much risk of misunderstanding or confusion of roles, but where there is a change of environment, or dramatic change in the pattern of management in the same environment, the professionals involved may become uneasy about their roles.

The anxiety expressed by nurses about the need for a strong medical line, partly illustrates the fact that we do not operate in a situation where each profession enjoys the same legal authority, but it also illustrates the anxiety of professionals about their accountability before the press, the public and the law courts. Collective responsibility and accountability is not yet recognised so each individual is left to stand on his own.

The opportunity for the team to criticise and evaluate its performance and the activities of its members, is not only necessary to improve the standard of patient care and to clarify individual roles, but is an important way of sharing responsibility and giving mutual support.

Third, where there is not adequate consultation and critical evaluation of the team's performance, there is danger of 'buck passing' and recriminations. The particular stresses in inter-professional relationships tend to appear when there are allegations of incompetence or professional misconduct, where in a situation demanding public accountability there tends to be a closing of the ranks, a denial of mistakes and blaming of other professional groups. The test of the viability of the inter-professional team is its capacity to cope with crises and failures—to share the blame, to accept responsibility and support the one who has had to make the decisions. This presupposes a degree of maturity and responsibility among those on the team which is the exception rather than the rule.

In the team where roles and responsibilties remain unclear there is likely to be 'buck passing' with 'difficult' or 'unco-operative' individuals, or with cases suggesting failure. There is at this point a conflict between the dependency of professionals on one another and their need for help, and the refusal to be the repository of the other's anxiety.

Specific areas of inter-professional conflict in relation to terminal care which were repeatedly mentioned in Working Group discussions were: disagreements about communicating prognoses, disagreements about medication and the level of sedation, about pain control, and about the allocation of time and resources.

The value and significance of the inter-professional case-conference. A variety of reasons were given for the consultant holding a case-conference and seeking a second opinion: i) the consultant could be seeking further information, wanting to be utterly sure of the facts (the declared reasons); ii) the consultant might be wanting to cover himself against legal comebacks; iii) he might be using the process of consultation as a substitute for taking a decision, or iv) he might be using it as a cover for testing out other people's attitudes and possible reactions (undeclared but important subsidiary motives), v) he might simply be using it as a means to communicate with his staff and thus achieve acceptance of his decision.

In this case the function of the case-conference was 'to arrest the spread of contagious indecision'. 'There had been a disturbance in the patterns of tacit agreement and authority. The case-conference was designed to restore cohesion to a disrupted group.' The explicit dilemmas were faced and a course of action decided upon. The case-conference also served as much as a means to defuse the tension as a means to reaching a consensus decision. It was also questioned whether it was used in this case primarily to reach a genuine consensus or as a contrivance to bolster the authority of the consultant. ('It was an authoritarian "consensus". There was no vigorous dissent.') The dilemmas concerned the choice of means not ends. There was no serious disagreement about ends (even the protest of the night nurse implied acceptance of the need to settle for comfort). Was the dilemma created by the consultant 'not positively being positive'? Ironically, the quick decision of the parents followed from their acceptance of the doctor's authority and expertise! The neglect of the parents showed that the true purpose and function of the case-conference was not to meet their need, but that of the anxious staff. 'What was tried was to achieve a consensus in an acute situation and it didn't work. Consensus is certainly better and more possible in slow care situations.'

The explicit reasons for and advantages of case-conferences were given as follows: i) to gather information and make use of skills and expertise from a variety of sources; ii) to generate discussion from outwith the unit (as in s w reports on home and family circumstances); and iii) to commit all staff to support the collective decision.

More indirect but important purposes served by case-conferences which were also mentioned were: i) they serve to contain the conflict between various interests in the inter-disciplinary team, allowing opportunity for the assertion of responsibility, recognition of competence and the sharing of responsibility. (By the same token they provide an opportunity for the manipulation of other staff and the creation of the illusion of consensus when what is sought is justification for a decision already made.) ii) Case-conferences can provide an opportunity for all involved in a crisis to come to terms with the irreducible elements of uncertainty and ambiguity with which decision-making is fraught.

Doubt was expressed as to whether the case-conference was a useful instrument for decision-making. With the diffuse and widening public expectations of the NHS, health-care teams were expected to decide on issues ranging from the narrowest clinical matters to the broadest issues of social welfare. In such situations individual professionals and particularly doctors tend understandably to be reticent to take decisions outwith the specific area of their professional competence. In such circumstances a case-conference could be a useful means of reaching a responsible consensus about what ought to be done, but would not necessarily help to decide who should take the initiative. In practice the willingness to take decisions often decided the issue in favour of the doctor—because it is not the ability to decide but the willingness to accept responsibility for a decision which usually decides the issue. However, the doctor might need the support of the team to enable him to take a decision or alternatively to delegate the authority to some other member of the team, while continuing to accept legal accountability for the decisions of the health-care team.

As a means for resolving moral dilemmas the case-conference was seen to have real value—particularly where the dilemmas in question appear to be structural, i.e. following from the disturbed pattern of institutional relationships. Here it can serve as a device for reappraisal of institutional arrangements, as a possible means of improving communication in institutional contexts, and as a means of expressing and thus creating new forms of intra- and inter-professional support. However, where more fundamental moral dilemmas arise—as in circumstances which seem to call for euthanasia—the case-conference is no more able to resolve the conflict of values involved than the individual professional is able to do on his own. The conflict of values in the case of a genuine dilemma cannot, *ex hypothesi*, be resolved by a decision of principle. The only way

139

may be to accept the unpleasant risk and responsibility of being wrong. Here the collective support and consensus of the team conference can help alleviate the anxiety, safeguard against the capricious action of individuals acting on their own, and indirectly protect the rights and interests of the patient. Where the choice is between two evils there may be no way to decide which is the lesser, but either to postpone a decision or to act and accept collective responsibility for a decision which may be wrong. Here the decision of the consultant to call a case-conference might have been construed as an evasion of responsibility on his part, or the most responsible thing he could do. The ambiguity remains. Where there is no consensus on the team the anxiety and tension can be considerable. If the doctor or someone else is not prepared to take a decision the only alternative is painful indecision, the polarisation of attitudes and prolonged crisis. Anxiety focuses on the likelihood of critical public reactions and the risk of legal action being taken.

The nature of values. We have not attempted to define professional values but have sought to illustrate what is understood in practice by professional values by providing a kind of definition-in-use of them. Both in the consideration of the case-material and in the subsequent discussion the question of the meaning of the term 'value' has not been raised directly but rather indirectly.

It is difficult to *say* what we mean by values for the term 'value' like the term 'meaning' is so basic to everyday discourse that it is either self-evidently obvious what we mean, or we have to stand back from ordinary usage and attempt second-order explanations of our first-order usage which involve us in the most abstract questions of philosophical logic, semantics and the metaphysics of value. We adopted the course throughout our study of having recourse to philosophical distinctions only when necessary and have attempted to *illustrate* the meanings of key terms rather than to define them.

In *Values in Social Work* the Working Party on the teaching of the value bases of social work offered the following useful description of the term 'value':

2.05 A value determines what a person thinks he *ought* to do, which may or may not be the same as what he wants to do, or what it is in his interest to do, or what in fact he actually does. Values in this sense give rise to general standards and ideals by which we judge our own and other's conduct; they also give rise to specific obligations.

This description is useful because it is fairly vague. In saying that values 'determine what a person thinks he ought to do' it does not specify how it is that values create this sense of obligation whether by widespread acceptance, divine authority or the force of moral

140

conviction. The detailed exploration of the relationship between values and obligations is the task of moral philosophy. In general we may say that what a man values he will strive for. The values which he endorses set the goals of his life and to some extent determine the steps he must take if he is to achieve his goals. To the extent that his values are self-chosen and self-imposed the duties or obligations which he must recognise are simply the conditions which he *must* fulfil if he is to succeed in achieving his goals and thus some realisation of his values. However, as the CCETSW publication emphasises, the term 'value' suggests something more than private tastes:

> 2.07   Values are distinguished from personal preferences in that they have been accepted and articulated to some degree by a group, of which the individual is probably a member. . . .
>
> 2.08   A value is used then as a socially accepted standard (at least by some group/s/) which guides the individual in the making of choices. . . .
>
> 2.09   A value can be operative only when the individual has knowledge of what he or she is doing, is aware of alternative courses of action and where there is a possibility of *choice* among these alternatives. . . .

Values thus are felt to have some degree of inter-personal validity in terms of which the individual judges his actions and by which his actions are judged by others—particularly those in the group with whom he shares the same values. The sense of obligation which commitment to a set of values gives to the individual is partly self-imposed, partly spelt out by the rules adopted by the community with whom he shares his values—as means for the realisation of their common ideals.

In discussing the values of particular professional groups it is obvious that at one and the same time Doctors, Nurses, Social Workers and Ministers (for example) share certain broad common humanitarian values, but that they also value particular kinds of knowledge and expertise which define the differences between their professional roles. The latter would to some extent be seen as the means for the realisation of the former. The knowledge of medicine, whether it be knowledge of physiology and pathology, the aetiology of diseases, or skills in diagnosis, surgery or the administration of drugs, each have their own value and could be pursued for their own sake, but they would normally be the instrumental means for the pursuit of more general values such as the service of suffering mankind. Likewise the special knowledge and skills of Nurses, Social Workers and Ministers serve to give specific content to the values of their professions, determining their professional roles and

L   141

duties. However, the caring functions of each of these professions tend to overlap in certain areas and this creates the possibility of conflict as they each variously interpret their duties in terms of their defined professional roles and functions.

The Working Group though aware of differences between the values of Doctors, Nurses, Social Workers and Ministers, expressed a considerable degree of agreement over the importance of the following values as basic to the caring professions: i) the ideal of truthfulness and openness in relationships based on confidentiality; ii) the ideal of facilitating the self-determination of the patient or client; iii) the ideal of acting as an advocate for those unable to defend their own interests in conflicts with other persons, professionals or institutions; iv) the ideal of providing continuity of care; v) the ideal of giving emergency help, treatment and care to the helpless and unconsultable individual.

If such general ideals were the only values determining professional conduct obviously there would not be major disagreements between different professionals. However it is equally clear that disagreements do arise but that they tend to arise at the level of the choice of means for the realisation of these ideals. Many dilemmas that arise in inter-professional relationships in practice relate more to problems of organisation and whether institutional arrangements for inter-professional communication are adequate or not. Disagreements about whether to communicate a bad prognosis do not compromise the ideal of truthfulness or openness, but tend to revolve around questions of how much should be told, at what stage and by whom. The right of the patient to know, if he demands to be told the truth, is an issue about which there may be theoretical disagreement, but the more common practical issue is who is the most acceptable or appropriate person to tell and how much responsibility should he be willing to accept to give continuing moral support to the patient afterwards. Such questions can only be decided by sensible and sensitive inter-professional consultation. Likewise on the subject of the sharing of confidential information between professions, it was recognised that the Nurses and Doctor can feel left out by the Social Worker or Minister, just as the Minister or Social Worker can feel excluded by the confidences of the medical staff. The issue of confidentiality thus often appears not as a strictly moral problem, but as a device by which the professional claims proprietorship of certain information as a means of retaining a hold over 'his' patients or clients and fending off other professionals:

More hokum is talked about confidentiality than anything else. After all whose confidences are they? The real question is: Is the client willing for the information to be passed on? When confidentiality matters it matters crucially, but more often than not people do not object to proper disclosure if it is in their best interests. Too often they are not asked or properly informed about what will be done with the information. Too often the appeal to confidentiality is just a means for one professional fencing off another.

If these examples serve to illustrate typical dilemmas in inter-professional relationships then they are fundamentally practical dilemmas raised by inadequate provision of means of communication and definition of professional roles in institutional settings. Even the religious justification given by the night nurse for her act of disobedience could be seen as forced upon her by a situation in which she was not adequately consulted or informed and not given adequate support in the exercise of her responsibilities. Clearly not all moral dilemmas are reducible to practical dilemmas, but it was felt that the majority of apparent moral dilemmas relate to problems of structure, organisation and communications in institutional work settings.

The case-conference is obviously no panacea, but only one device for attempting to improve inter-professional communication and the clarification of roles which is a *sine qua non* for effective decision-making in inter-professional contexts. In so far as professional values are institutionalised in professional roles, the clarification of roles is thus both a way of safeguarding and affirming professional values. The fear that professional values will be compromised or rejected in inter-professional team co-operation is not borne out in practice. If anything the contrary is true. The experience of good inter-professional co-operation tends to confirm the identity and dignify the separate functions of each participating professional. The competitive element in inter-professional relationships may well sharpen up some of the differences between doctors, nurses, social workers and ministers but equally well it reminds members of each profession of the many values they have in common as members of the 'caring professions'.

SUGGESTED READING FOR CHAPTER EIGHT

The studies listed in the Bibliography under British Medical Association (1974), Central Council (1976), Eadie (1975), Emmet (1966), Freidson (1970), Goode (1960), International Council of Nurses (1965 and 1973), Mackay (1976), Mitchell (1976), Parsons (1951 and 1954), Royal College of Nursing (1976), Thompson (1976).
Values, Professional Ethics and the Social Worker: Bernstein

(1960), Biestek (1957), Briar & Miller (1972), Central Council (1976), Emmet (1967), Foren & Bailey (1968), Goldstein (1973), Halmos (1965), Hollis (1967), Irvine (1964), Keith-Lucas (1963), Timms (1970), Wardron (1957).

Values, Professional Ethics and the Nursing Profession: Anderson (1973), Bady (1973), Hockey (1976), MacLean (1974).

Values, Professional Ethics and the Ministry: Blackham, Brothers (1971), Eadie (1972, 1973, 1974), Ference *et al.* (1971), Hill (1973), Jarvis (1976), Martin (1967), Milton (1972).

Medical References: Balint (1957), Cartwright (1967), Cronin (1937), Ferris (1965 and 1967), Fraser *et al.* (1976), Friedson (1975), Lewis and Maud (1952), McKeown (1965), Miller (1973), Nuffield Provincial Hospitals Trust (1972), Pappworth (1967), Poynter (1969), Poynter (1971), Stevens (1966).

IN   aced by pro-
fe: anxiety was
ex   rement. The
m(: i) whether
bei   as an illness: ii) the danger of
medicalising bereavement; iii) the problems faced by the professional confronted with the over-demanding chronically bereaved
individual; and iv) where to draw the limits to professional responsibility in caring for the bereaved.

The case presented concerns a woman who suffered a severe but
perhaps not atypical bereavement. The husband and GP had kept
from her the seriousness of his heart condition. The widow's depression, self-neglect and 'morbid' desire to die led relatives to put pressure on the GP to give her anti-depressant drugs and finally to have
her admitted to a psychiatric hospital where she was given further
drug treatment and ECT. After eighteen months, with two brief re-
missions, she was still receiving treatment as a psychiatric out-
patient.

Views on the appropriate nature and scope of professional, and
particularly medical, involvement in the care of the bereaved were
divided on the basis of different personal 'philosophies' and ideals
of service. Consequently the chapter concludes with three personal
statements, by a GP, a Hospital Doctor and a Nurse, outlining their
respective views on their responsibilities to the bereaved. These are
included because they represent three different approaches to the
ideal of caring involvement by doctors and nurses with the bereaved.

Professional Involvement in the Care of the Bereaved

There was a general reluctance to accept that problems of
bereavement are the responsibility of medical and nursing staff as
well as of the minister and social worker. It was recognised that the
general practitioner and district nurse have certain responsibilities
to follow up bereaved relatives and that in the cases of pathological

grief reactions the psychiatrist may become involved. There remained a general inhibition in the Group to discuss the problems of bereavement. To professionals, trained to maintain an attitude of affective neutrality, the emotional stresses of bereavement present disconcerting problems. The professional may have difficulty coming to terms with his own bereavement where the relationship between professional and client has been a long-standing and significant one. He is reluctant to get involved in the taxing and emotionally demanding situation of caring for the bereaved, or having to cope with the emotional distress and conflict. However, personal experience of bereavement influences professional attitudes profoundly. Those who had personally experienced the loss of a close relative emphasised the need to give attention to the care and support of the bereaved, and were more willing to give that support themselves.

In general, doctors and nurses, but also social workers and ministers, receive inadequate training in the handling of the problems of bereavement. This results in failure to recognise the bereavement of the dying patient himself, and his need for support in facing the loss of life and separation from the family and friends; and is related to inadequate training in the communication of bad prognoses and such essential practical procedures as the communication of death messages. General ignorance of the patterns of normal and pathological grief-reactions leaves professionals uncertain how to respond and how to deal appropriately with the bereaved. The recent studies of bereavement by Murray Parkes, Elizabeth Kübler-Ross, Lily Pincus and others were welcomed, as well as the growing awareness among professionals of the problems of bereavement and of their role in giving care and support.

Concern was expressed at the vast expansion of professional responsibility which undertaking support for the bereaved implies in practice for doctors and nurses, but also for other professionals. How can the professional set reasonable limits to his involvement with the bereaved when grief-states can be very protracted and the bereaved can become very demanding? Hospital doctors and nurses were concerned about the limited amount which they could do to help. General practitioners and nurses accepted that they have increasing responsibility to care for the bereaved in the aftermath of a death, but were uncertain about the proper extent of their continuing involvement after the first months. Social workers, ministers and psychiatrists recognised that their help tends to be required when the problems of grief are protracted or manifest pathological symptoms but were concerned about the problems of dependency created by their longer-term professional involvement.

Doubts were expressed about whether bereavement ought to be a medical or professional responsibility. It was recognised that with medical advance and the changing pattern of morbidity, with an increasing proportion of deaths among the elderly and isolated, the medical and allied professions have inherited responsibility for the care of the bereaved. This fairly recent development was linked with social changes which have come about with the transition to an increasingly urban and industrial society, the greater mobility of people and the breakdown of the extended family and the traditional community support for the bereaved. The accompanying privatisation of death and bereavement (Boyd, K.M., 1977) has led to an increased proportion of hospital deaths and to a growing demand for professional help in times of grief and loss. The decline in church attendance and support for official religion has meant that the ministry of the clergy has been less relied on with a corresponding increase in dependence on the general practitioner (as the professional most readily available and able to provide continuity of care). To a lesser extent people have also come to depend on social workers, the psychiatric services and voluntary agencies to provide the help once provided by the family, the minister and the community. It was doubted that these trends could be reversed and therefore it was accepted that in the future there will necessarily be increasing pressure on professionals to become involved in care and support of the bereaved.

Finally, the well documented evidence of increased mortality and morbidity among the bereaved (Parkes, C.M., 1976, and Rees, W.D. and Lutkins, S.G., 1967) (whether bereavement makes people illness-prone or simply exposes the latent morbidity of the individuals concerned), was taken as sufficient justification for medical intervention in the care of the bereaved — at least in terms of a responsibility for the doctor to maintain adequate surveillance and follow-up of affected relatives. However, there was a general feeling that the tendency for bereavement to be seen as a problem requiring medical or professional help may be unfortunate as it may lead to the medicalisation of what should be a natural process.

The tendency for bereavement to be treated as an illness was seen to have advantages to the bereaved themselves, in helping them to accept the often bizarre physical and psychological reactions associated with acute grief and in helping to legitimise their approach to doctors and other members of the caring professions for help. However, there were seen to be dangers implicit in the acceptance of bereavement as 'a temporary psychological illness', for this discouraged people from learning to cope with their loss and encouraged them to see themselves as sick instead. The double risk of this medicalisation of the problem is that by encouraging the bereaved to adopt the patient role it encourages attitudes of dependency and puts pressure on the professional to treat the bereaved individual as someone who requires drugs, or psychiatric treatment, or special social assistance. To the extent that the bereaved is made into a patient or treated as a helpless and inadequate individual, professional involvement with the bereaved becomes counterproductive and imposes excessive demands and responsibilities on the professional.

Both psychiatrists and social workers emphasised the value of seeing the responses of the individual to bereavement against the background of general human responses to loss. Psychiatrists emphasised that the individual's capacity to cope with the loss of a loved one tends to be related to their experiences of rejection, abandonment and loss during childhood and adult life and how they learned to cope with these. Social workers stressed the analogies to bereavement in the experiences of families having to part with children into care, in the breakdown of a marriage and divorce, and in facing redundancy and loss of status. This emphasis on loss and reaction to loss was seen as useful to the professional in explaining the nature of individual responses to bereavement, and as useful to the bereaved in emphasising that the experience of loss is inescapable in life and that we have to learn to come to terms with it.

The emphasis on bereavement as a challenge and opportunity for growth was emphasised by bereaved persons involved in voluntary self-help organisations for the bereaved, and emphasised by ministers and psychiatrists. The value of this approach was seen in the fact that it encouraged individuals to begin again, to help themselves and to look outside themselves for sources of faith and hope for living. Its limitations are that by itself it does not sufficiently emphasise the very real need and dependency of the bereaved at certain stages of bereavement, that it does not take seriously the extent to which the bereaved may be genuinely ill, and that it does not take full account of the reality and depth of the experience of bereavement in its own terms.

None of these models of bereavement is adequate in itself, and only those who have suffered bereavement and its physical and psychological effects can affirm to what degree it is an illness, an experience of loss with a unique and shattering finality, of having to grow painfully and slowly towards a new hope that life can begin again. The value of these different models was seen in terms of providing different ways in which professionals could understand their various roles in the care of the bereaved.

Case presentation, by a Psychiatrist

This case was used as a basis for the case-conference because it was felt to raise all the previously identified dilemmas about bereavement. Though an example of a rather severe bereavement reaction it was not felt to be atypical. The Working Group agreed that there is increasing pressure on GPs to prescribe drugs for bereavement and to make psychiatric referrals if grief states are severe. The ambiguity of this case, however, provided occasion for much discussion and disagreement.

'Mrs A.' aged 62

I was called to see this lady by her family doctor. She had returned from her sister's house three weeks previously and had been depressed throughout this time. She sits at home, staring into space. She doesn't eat even the food her neighbours give her. She had been like this most of the time since her husband's death four months ago. She frequently says she wishes she were dead. Her sister had visited for two days and had made it clear to the GP that 'something had to be done' before she could leave her to return to her own family in England. The GP added that anti-depressant drugs had not had any effect, and requested admission.

When I visited the home she was sitting motionless in a spotless but cold house. Her sister said she was like that all the time, and wouldn't even bother to go to bed, cook and put on the fire when she wasn't around. Her husband, who had been a brewery worker, had died unexpectedly a few months after his retirement. It transpired that he and the doctor knew he had angina but it had been kept from her. The marriage of 30 years' duration had been 'happy but they had no children'. They were quiet and respected in the neighbourhood without being well known to anyone. All agreed that they were very dependent on each other. They did not go to church. His principal interest was music and he had just been given a Hi Fi as a retirement present which she couldn't bear to look at. She wanted them 'to take it away again quickly'. Immediately after the funeral she had gone to stay with her sister in England whose husband had coped with 'all the arrangements'. Her profound depression, silence, refusal to eat and talk of suicide had caused her relatives to call their doctor, and a psychiatrist had admitted her to a mental hospital where she received anti-depressants and ECT. She was much 'better' after one month—talkative, active and asked to go home to her sister. This improvement persisted until she came to live on her own in Edinburgh, when she swiftly declined.

As she was on her own and there seemed to be suicidal risk coupled with community pressure to have her admitted, she came without opposition into hospital. I regarded her as suffering from a profound grief reaction and we hoped that exploration of this would enable her to return home. Conventional methods to help her to express her grief and talk about her past proved fruitless, as did abreaction which was later tried. She was in hospital for more than six months (I had originally anticipated two to three weeks). Eventually she was given a range of anti-depressant drugs and improved markedly.

She returned to her house for progressively longer periods and seemed quite at ease. She no longer talked of getting rid of the house and could recognise and accept her grief. The social worker and health visitor kept in regular touch and the local church was also enlisted to involve her in the area. After three months at home she was invited on holiday to her sister.

At this point I lost touch until I received a letter two weeks ago from the psychiatrist in England saying that she had been in hospital for a further period and was now improved. She was returning to Edinburgh soon, and he wondered if I would undertake her 'out-patient' supervision. Approximately nine of the eighteen months since her husband's death have been spent in hospital—she has no history of previous psychiatric illness.

Illustrative discussion

The first major issue discussed concerned the difficulties which arise in inter-professional communication because doctors, nurses and other health-care professionals do not anticipate the needs of the bereaved and are uncertain about their role in the care of the bereaved. The possible role of nurses and doctors in preparing relatives for bereavement requires inter-professional co-operation and the sharing of relevant information between all members of the team.

Ward Sister. Why aren't nurses told more about the family circumstances of patients, as well as the medical details of the case? Without some idea of the prognosis and the needs of the family, nurses are inadequately prepared to help the patient or the family and others closely involved.

GP. It is only with hindsight that you say more social background would have helped. How can the hospital sister help prepare relatives for bereavement? Surely this is more the responsibility of the GP?

Ward Sister. If the GP passes on adequate information to the hospital staff it greatly facilitates their communication with patient and family. You have a better overall understanding of the feelings in a family if you know their circumstances.

GP. I would question this. Lack of information provides an opportunity to ask, to explore, to enquire. Giving knowledge in an encapsulated form may be a barrier to personal involvement.

Ward Sister. If two ward sisters and five staff nurses all ask the patient the same questions it is useless and frustrating to the patient. Patients get impatient with repetitive enquiries. Knowing some basic facts (e.g. whether the patient and/or relatives know the prognosis) enables nurses to avoid doing negative things. If you know something about them in advance you can welcome them and show genuine concern in this case.

Psychiatrist. There is often a feeling of the nurse being on her own in relation to the rest of the team. There is a case for developing a place for management of death and bereavement in the way a hospital team plans for an operation. There is no serious team discussion of appropriate information for the anticipation of the problems of the bereaved. That this woman didn't know her husband had angina or the likely prognosis was certainly a complicating factor in her bereavement.

Ward Sister. If the nurses know that a situation is terminal there is a lot they can do to help which has a bearing on later bereavement. They can bend the rules regarding visiting, encourage relatives to assist in small ways with nursing and feeding for example, make opportunities for patients and relatives to have the privacy necessary to work out together some of their anticipatory grief, and be more available to meet enquiries and to discuss things with patients and relatives.

The 'conspiracy of silence' surrounding death, has an effect on subsequent bereavement and its management. The effect of being cut off from her husband and the doctor over so important a matter as his potentially fatal heart condition, left Mrs A. unprepared for her subsequent bereavement and also complicated the subsequent management of her bereavement. Because the doctor did not see her as part of his responsibility, and did not give her the opportunity to discuss things with him, she may well have had to present as someone in need of medical and psychiatric treatment in order to get the care she needed. The unwillingness of medical and nursing staff to see care of the bereaved as part of their responsibility may, paradoxically, lead to the medicalisation of bereavement—as people present with various psycho-somatic complaints and demand drugs and tranquillisers instead of being able to seek support and opportunity to talk out their problems with the doctor or other professionals.

Medical involvement with the bereaved. The pathology of bereavement is to some extent society-induced: the bereaved are isolated in their grief, produce the external signs of distress, then society pressurises the G P and the psychiatrist to treat the symptomatic effects produced by this isolation rather than give people the time and opportunity to talk out their grief. Increased morbidity and mortality among widows and widowers means that the doctor, partly because of his ready availability, is required to provide *some* kind of care for the bereaved. Whether he is prepared to give time for ventilatory discussion or has recourse to drugs depends to some extent on his role and responsibilities and his willingness to act out a different role with the person concerned rather than treat them as a patient.

Chaplain. Increasingly people turn to the doctor for help with their bereavement. This also means increasing dependency of people on G Ps and Hospital Doctors. To what extent, one might ask, do they encourage this dependency? How do we explain the customary valium left on the mantlepiece? As a parish minister I found this was very common. It seemed that doctors didn't want to go through the painful experience of tears, grief, etc. and to prescribe Valium was the way out.

GP. Regarding the Valium on the mantlepiece . . . People have long had recourse to alcohol to help them get over their grief. Valium may have become a socially acceptable alternative, and a necessary aid in the absence of means such as the traditional 'wake' for the collective sharing of grief.

An admitted disadvantage of Valium may be in relation to 'grief work', drugs may simply postpone the pain and delay the necessary process of grieving and grief-work. I believe funerals are desirable in helping people get over their grief and isolation. In our society it is still acceptable to show outward signs of grief at funerals. It also brings the bereaved into contact with other people again. Many disapprove of the ritual of shaking hands after the funeral, but one point in its favour is that it helps the bereaved to get over the break, forces them into meeting people.

Chaplain. But it doesn't help when they are so heavily sedated that they don't know what's going on—as is often the case.

Physician. But the reasons for recourse to Valium are also more non-specific. It arises out of popular beliefs regarding things like regular bowel movements—that a good night's sleep is imperative. All too often we read of a child burnt in some house accident, and the mother put on sedatives. It arises out of a belief that the worst possible thing that can happen is to lose a night's sleep. There is a good deal of anxiety about insomnia and demand for sedatives.

2nd SW. On the other hand the bereaved are usually occupied during the day. It is a question of being strung up and alone at night, often unused to being alone. The answer may be for the daughter to come and stay, but where no such arrangement is possible, the Valium may be of help.

Hospital Doctor. Shouldn't we ask whether the suppression of grief and anxiety is dysfunctional?

Social Worker. It is a matter of professional response and responsibility. It arises out of a situation where you are expected to do something, where you want to do something, but you don't know what the appropriate response is. You feel called upon to make a professional response—however, to prescribe Valium may not be the most responsible thing to do.

GP. Yes. This is an important area of moral dilemma—how to respond to pressure as a professional.

Physician. I'd like to ask whether bereavement is really a medical matter at all? Like care of the dying, care of the bereaved seems to have become a medical matter by inheritance. We just stand by waiting for the community to come roaring in, but they don't. Does bereavement make you ill? Or does loss of a spouse and grief expose existing illness and weakness? Murray Parkes cannot be taken at face value—let us remember that most of the sick are elderly and most dying is done by old people!'

2nd SW. It is not only bereavement which exposes the morbidity of the aged, but any kind of major shock or change. It can be the separation of husband and wife when one is sent off to hospital, or even going away on holiday, or moving house.

Hospital Doctor. Is there a tendency towards the medicalisation of bereavement?

Psychiatrist. The immediate effect of a death is different from the reaction a couple of days later. Do we give Valium to placate the relatives? There is a difference here between the way that young and old people cope with grief. Often young people are less likely to want extravagant expressions of grief, are afraid of it and ask for Valium to keep the widow quiet. Where does the profession stand in relation to this problem? In general there are no contra-indications, on the medical evidence, for prescribing Valium for the first 6 hours. However, barbiturates for the whole course of a bereavement can be devastating. This is the area where there is risk of medicalisation. The dilemma is how to respond to social pressure.

SW. Does 'prescribing' something have a symbolic value here? Is it the doctor's way of expressing caring?

153

Physician. It is a question of to what extent medical intervention can be justified.

2nd SW. There may be value to the bereaved in speaking of bereavement as an 'illness'. It is a process to be suffered and gone through, and there may be need for medication and special caring.

Physician. Abnormal reactions justify medical intervention, but has the doctor anything to offer that could not be provided by a minister? Has he a special medical charisma which can help here?

GP. Bereavement is not necessarily an illness, though traumatic shock and grief are inherently abnormal. We must distinguish between the physical and psychological symptoms which are the normal concommitants of grief, and pathological symptoms. Is helping those with 'normal' bereavement doing anything more than acting as a good neighbour? The doctor is someone who can help by explaining the physical and psychological developments. He can help by encouraging patients to ventilate their anxieties about such things as hallucinations and fears of delusion or madness.

Hospital Doctor. The doctor's role is one of education and/or management in the bereavement phase.

It was questioned whether there is any standard or 'appropriate' professional response to bereavement—because reactions to death and bereavement are so varied. In general it was felt that the best that could be advocated was a caring response based on flexibility according to needs and available resources, remembering that often the kindest form of care is professional efficiency. In most circumstances there is limited time, and attention has to be concentrated on efficient action and functional communication directed towards help with immediate practical problems.

The limits of professional involvement

Reverting to the case of Mrs A., it was suggested that she illustrated the problem of those lacking the intermediate support of family and friends (i.e. between her GP and voluntary mutual-help organisations like CRUSE, she had no one to whom she could turn). In her case medical treatment was started too early and the medicalisation of her bereavement began with the GP's anxiety that from being a capable and independent woman prior to her husband's death she was at risk of becoming a chronic dependent. His anxiety and haste to see her over her bereavement paradoxically confirmed her in a dependent role, thus making it more difficult in turn for the doctor to withdraw.

GP. In the case of Mrs A. the psychiatrist did all that was open to him and most helpfully. On the indications, the administration of anti-depressants and even ECT was probably justified. It is doubtful whether this is a case of unjustified medicalisation of a bereavement. At any rate, at the time that the patient was referred to him it is doubtful that he could have done otherwise than he did.

Chairman. Do you have a boundary line as a person, or as a doctor?

GP. You are involved as a doctor in the immediate bereavement, then there is the follow-up after the funeral, then you let people come to you. I don't think one is being effective as a doctor if one encourages 'My old doctor was a friend of the family' kind of attitude. One must keep it on a professional level, and bereave as a doctor!

Nurse. CRUSE know what normal grieving is and as widows give a great deal of help to those going through it. They also know how to recognise those who need medical help and can distinguish from personal experience between normal and abnormal grief. I have learned a lot from them. They know how to get involved and when to withdraw. Mrs A. should have been put in touch with CRUSE once no more treatment could be given her. The professional with personal experience of bereavement may also find it easier to know how much or how little he should get involved in a particular case.

Physician. The doctor's own grief or remorse that things have not gone as he had planned, have not gone right at the end, can also determine the degree of responsibility he feels and the extent of his continuing involvement with relatives — both positively and negatively.

GP. The doctor must be more aware, alert to the early signs of morbidity, that's good preventive medicine. Increasing morbidity is not an affront — but the natural way of nature. In practice he should withdraw early, but be available if needed. He should not intervene directly.

Psychiatrist. What do you do about the chronic bereaved?

SW. Or the chronic dependent for whom bereavement is a pretext?

Chaplain. It depends to some extent on your view of the scope and limits of your professional role, and your personal ideals of service, as well as willingness to accept the limits of your own strength and resources, and personal need for help in coping.

Comment and personal statements

It was generally agreed that the tendency towards the medicalisation of bereavement is unfortunate and that it is better to seek community help for the bereaved. Professional knowledge and expertise should be used to mobilise and create means of community support, to educate lay people in the facts of bereavement and to facilitate them and voluntary organisations to play a more effective part in dealing with the problems of the bereaved.

Attitudes of different members of the Working Group to the nature and scope of their responsibilities were clearly related to their personal experience of grief and mourning, views of their own profession and its ideals, and their own moral and religious beliefs. Because there was considerable diversity of attitude and belief about these matters it was felt to be appropriate that some examples should be given to illustrate how different personal philosophies give rise to different views of the ideal caring involvement of doctors and nurses with the bereaved. Consequently three personal statements, by a Houseman, Senior Nurse and General Practitioner, are given below to illustrate this conclusion of the Working Group rather than analytical comment.

A HOUSEMAN'S view. There are essentially three phases in the relationship between houseman and the bereaved.

The first meeting is the day of admission or soon after. This is an important meeting as I introduce myself in name and manner. The meeting also allows me to meet the relatives and assess them in terms of intelligence, background, fears and hopes. I often form a general view of the prognosis by the time I have clerked the patient into the ward and I present this general view to the relatives at this first meeting. 'Things don't look too good, but we have tests to do' or 'She is an old lady and they don't stand up to these things as easily as you or me.'

I take great care at this first meeting not to suggest a plan of management, but to await their reply and reaction. They have sometimes assessed the picture correctly. 'We knew she was very ill. She has never been the same since Dad died.' 'Poor old soul, she has had no life for some time now.' Sometimes they don't receive it well, become upset and demand dates, times and a rigid agenda of expected progress of the disease. 'How long has he got?' 'Will you operate soon?'

I find it is important not to give way and provide information which later will be proved wrong. I try to listen and let them talk. Occasionally aggression may be expressed at this time or anger about other doctors. 'I told our own doctor he was unwell but he kept giving him tablets and a sick line.' I take care again not to agree or disagree but to listen. I feel this is often an expression of guilt on the relatives' part that they themselves did not do enough.

The second phase is when results of biopsies, operation or other tests are available. Between the two phases I try to keep contact with relatives, but try not to spend too long with them as it only raises hopes that I have something new to tell them. As soon as the results are through I arrange a meeting and clearly, and in language that is understandable to them, give them the firm diagnosis and probable outcome. They often accept this more easily as a lot of the initial aggression, fears and reservations have been expressed at the first meeting. They often make it clear that they do or do not want the patient to be told. 'I don't want him to know', or 'I think he knows all is lost'. At this time I try to stress that what the patient wants is important and that their relationships are vitally important at this time. 'Is it not unfair at the time he most needs you that you both are separated by a dreadful secret?' As a result of support and talking with relatives earlier objections are often withdrawn.

Again the question of time is brought up. 'How long has he got?' I always evade answering this as I feel it imposes a great strain on all concerned. If the time is exceeded they build themselves up again for another date, which does not come, and so it goes on. If they don't reach the time limit then there is guilt that maybe they did not do every thing possible, etc. At any rate we are so often wrong.

The patient may remain ill in the ward and die, or go home only to be readmitted in a terminal state for care. I always see the relatives at the time of this admission and use first names and personal details as appropriate. I feel it is very important not to perform routine tests, e.g. haemoglobin, urea and electrolytes, unless it is used for action, e.g. blood transfusion, as this only causes confusion in relatives' minds that perhaps there is something more that can be done and causes discomfort for the patient.

When the patient dies I write the death certificate. In consultation with my seniors a decision is made about a post mortem. I see the relatives and generally arrange to have a cup of tea with them. I state plainly the fact that the patient has died and the cause of death. Initially I say very little letting them cry or talk without interruption. Then I show them the death certificate and explain what it means. I advise them about registration and answer the odd question about viewing of the body, disposing of the remains, etc. I then go over the illness and death in summary form. 'She had a long hard fight with the cancer. She is at peace now. She died peacefully. At least she was in no pain.' I hope they have been there when the patient died and that it was peaceful. I ask about the spouse and the rest of the family and who will look after them.

Questions are often raised about early management of the illness and I try to stem any feelings of guilt they may have at that time or are likely to have in the future. If they cry a lot I sit and touch them.

If a PM is required I broach the topic and try to put it as gently as possible. 'We would like an examination of the body.' I have never had any trouble with this but hate the job intensely.

Following this, I touch them and say cheerio. I am occasionally asked by relatives for drugs for the husband or spouse. I always refuse and say that time heals, and that their own doctor is the best person to give tablets as required. I then phone the GP and tell him the nature and cause of death and if a PM is proposed. In general I never see the relatives again.

The SENIOR STAFF NURSE stressed surprise at discovering that nurses have considerable contact with bereavement and opportunities to give support and practical help to the bereaved. Nurses meet bereavement in the course of routine nursing duties and are not merely involved in giving support to the relatives as an extension of their professional responsibilities to the dying patient. Instances mentioned were mothers with still births, the bereavement of other patients in long-stay wards when one of their number dies, the bereavement of survivors of road traffic accidents where relatives have been killed, and the particular problems of bereavement among the mentally handicapped, where it is assumed that patients 'don't understand'. She emphasised that nurses need to have impressed on them the extent of loss in bereavement and the fact that it is permissible and sometimes proper to grieve with patients. Also that nurses need opportunities to face and talk about their own experiences of bereavement. Finally, that nurses need to realise the opportunities there are on visits and at other times for educating and preparing about-to-be bereaved relatives. The Staff Nurse said:

Although nurses have become much more aware of their contribution to the care of the dying, on the whole they have not begun to appreciate the needs of the bereaved or to identify the relevant areas of nursing concern. Bereaved people are not 'ill' and usually are not 'patients'. Apart from the brief, immediate, post-death contact, nurses in hospital have no further responsibility for the bereaved. Even the community nurses who have been looking after a dying patient at home end their formal contact with the family after the death. However, despite this, nurses *do* become involved with bereaved people in a variety of

158

situations. Both in hospital and community settings, the nurse caring for a dying patient is inevitably involved with his family and visitors and support for these 'to-be-bereaved' people should be a natural extension of care of the patient. The post-death contact with the deceased's close relatives is a brief but significant involvement of the nurse in hospital, and one to which more attention should be given.

Also from time to time, patients in a hospital ward may have suffered a bereavement—for example, an elderly widow, the survivor of a multiple accident, a mother who has lost her new-born baby, or a patient in a psychiatric ward suffering from reactive depression. In any long-stay ward, some patients will be bereaved following the death of a co-patient. The effect of death on the ward on other patients is an issue to which nurses should give more attention, and generally the management of this kind of bereavement merits more serious consideration by medical and nursing staff. In the community, the DN or HV is bound to be involved with families who are bereaved.

It is sad that many nurses seem to feel that it is not 'professional' to be compassionate in an overt way. Being kind and considerate to visitors of a dying patient is a simple but essential way of giving support and compensating for some of the rather impersonal aspects of hospital care. Practical help can be invaluable for the family caring for a dying person at home, in particular teaching the relatives to cope with basic physical problems and providing essential equipment to do so. Advice about visiting in hospital can allay anxieties and providing as much privacy as possible for visits is essential. Listening to the fears and worries of the relatives can be revealing and the nurse can help to explain information given by the doctor and spend time talking about seemingly trivial worries which relatives feel the doctor is too busy to discuss. Preparing relatives for the practicalities of bereavement is also helpful, for example discussing in advance of the death how the relatives wish to be informed of the event and what they need to do immediately afterwards. In their contact with bereaved people in the longer term, nurses can provide support by making time to listen and discuss problems and in doing this acknowledge that the process of bereavement is a long and painful business.

Perhaps nurses would become better able to help bereaved people if they acknowledged their personal sense of loss when a patient dies. It is common practice to 'tidy away' a death in the ward, and to hide any emotional reactions. Expressing and sharing grief may not seem 'professional' but it is probably essential

159

and may be the only way for nurses to begin to recognise that bereavement is a natural process which can be better understood and coped with if it is shared with others.

The GENERAL PRACTITIONER referred to the possible opportunities of the family doctor to be both doctor and friend to the bereaved family. In the case where the bereaved relatives were also his patients he emphasised that the doctor has an obligation to give what friendly support he can and not be just a dispenser of drugs. He also suggested that the doctor should be sensitive to the spiritual needs of people at such times and while co-operating with the minister should not be embarrassed to share his own faith with the bereaved if it was appropriate. He emphasised that while his proposals represented an ideal they were not counsels of perfection, but seriously considered practical suggestions.

The problems and challenges of bereavement frequently start before the actual death. Close relatives have often been told of the expected outcome many months or years before this, and had to bear this knowledge alone or with close friends, but seldom with the patient himself. At this stage they carry an immense burden, being anxious to protect the patient (whom they usually think has no knowledge or understanding of the diagnosis or prognosis), anxious to do all possible for them, often unaware of the form the final illness will take and the physical and emotional difficulties and complications they will encounter, and yet often not prepared to admit to most of their feelings and fears lest it surprise their doctor or alert their loved one. The GP. said:

The second stage is that suffered at the time of the death itself, the features of which are well known and documented. This is followed by the immediate post-death phase lasting for 3-6 months during which the bereaved person attempts to gather his thoughts together, make plans for a new form of life and make a brave face for the world which by even 3 months seems to expect 'normality' and an end to 'grief'. The final stage is found in the years that follow when not only friends and relations but frequently the doctor expect that the suffering and re-adjustment are over and the loss of their loved one need not be referred to again.

Unlike many other professional helpers the general practitioner has many roles in this caring process. Whilst at all times he must maintain his professional role, that of the specially-trained scientific adviser, he must remain a 'friend', someone who, in the eyes of the bereaved, can shed his white coat image and be the one sitting by the fireside with a cup of coffee in his hands, ready to listen to anything that seems to matter to the patient, ready to share and understand, ready to proffer help. The uniqueness of this role is challenging yet difficult, and has to be seen as a great privilege given to few people today.

He wears more caps than these though. From the day that the patient is first informed of the diagnosis and ultimate prognosis the general practitioner may have to be an educator, explaining medical procedures, tests and operations, acting as an interpreter for hospital colleagues and, on many occasions, playing the role of co-ordinator bringing in different caring agencies and support services, restraining colleagues from over-enthusiastic intervention or interference, and often being responsible for bringing members of the family together so that all may share the burden and assist in whatever way is possible. Throughout this time he keeps a watching eye on their health, aware of the strains and suppressed fears and passions, mindful of their own medical history and its relevance in the light of known personality traits.

Unobtrusively, his own personal faith should be apparent and can be of enormous help to such patients though an opportunity to talk about it may never present itself. Patients frequently want to talk of spiritual matters, even their own loss of a previously meaningful faith, their guilt feelings in respect of such loss, their anxieties about a future life, the possible place of prayer, the comfort that a living faith seems to bring to others, and often what faith means to the doctor himself. It is often the dying one who first opens the subject, and then mentions this to their relatives who, in their turn, seek an oppprtunity to take the doctor on one side and 'casually' mention their minister or need for Church friendship before admitting that they are eager to talk of faith itself.

In the case of many Catholic families, so well supported by their priest, the eagerness is made easier by the encounters between doctor and priest when visiting the patient and his family.

These different but completely complementary roles of professional adviser, co-ordinator, physician, spiritual supporter, educator and friend are all played out in different degrees during each stage already mentioned in this paper.

Initially he can see himself as the 'preparer' for what is to come. Careful preparation can lessen the eventual problems though never the loss and loneliness. At the time of the death he is likely to be the only non-family person there, the only one not rent by sorrow, doubts, personal regrets and reproach, not tormented by anger. In addition to his statutory duties in certifying death he can give practical advice on the many practical matters that must be dealt

Case Studies in Moral Dilemmas

with, most of which are foreign to those intimately involved that day, matters that worry and sometimes terrify relatives.

After this 'death visit' I personally visit again on the day before the funeral and again a few days after, as much as anything to remind them of my presence and care for them rather than to diagnose or prescribe. They have to be shown, very clearly, that though their loved one has gone and no longer needs my care, they, the relatives left behind, are still my patients, still important to me, still deserving of every skill I may have even though they may have proved poor nurses, may have expressed anger and resentment towards me and other doctors, and may now be showing the weaker sides of their characters and personalities.

I then visit after about 3 weeks when family members have left for their scattered homes and the bereaved ones have protested that they can 'cope' perfectly well, and again see them, at home usually, or occasionally in the surgery, at 6 weeks and 12 weeks — both being times when serious emotional and physical breakdown start to show. At 6 months I offer a very full physical and emotional assessment to them, reminding them that their bereavement takes a toll on them of which even they may be unaware. This reminds them that they are not alone, not forgotten or neglected.

While increasing attention is being given to the subject of bereavement in courses for Social Workers and Ministers, not nearly enough time is devoted to bereavement in the training of doctors and nurses. Certain kinds of learning about bereavement are not readily taught but depend upon the experience and maturity of the individual and opportunities for sharing experience with other professionals in the work situation in the hospital or community. However, many simple things can be taught—e.g. about learning to listen, to appear concerned and unhurried, learning to touch people or hold their hand or speak less formally. More difficult is learning to be responsive to the needs of individuals—'You have to wait for their invitation. People offer you the privilege of greater intimacy. Do we accept the invitation and accept the responsibility that goes with it?' There is need for the creation of more obvious means of support for professionals involved with the bereaved and doctors, nurses, social workers and ministers need to be taught to examine their own attitudes to death and bereavement more critically, for unless they explore what they are afraid of and how they react themselves to grief and loss there is risk that their own attitudes will prevent them from dealing effectively with the situation.

The needs of the bereaved represent a challenge to the idealism of the professionals. To the medical and nursing profession it represents the challenge to reconcile the science of medicine with the art of proper health-care, the challenge to reconcile the limited and more technical responsibilities of the curative functions of medicine with the more unlimited and demanding responsibilities of care in the broadest sense. To the social workers and minister it represents a challenge to the role of counsellor and helper, namely the demand to be a more patient listener and the willingness to be involved over a long period in such a way that the bereaved person is neither patronised nor turned into a dependent. To all professionals bereavement represents the challenge to learn the skills required to facilitate bereaved persons to face their problems, renew their sources of faith and hope and have the courage to begin again.

SUGGESTED READING FOR CHAPTER NINE
The studies listed in the Bibliography under Bellis (1977), Boyd (1977), Black (1976), Carlson (1970), Contact (1964), Dewi Rees, Gibson (1974), Illich (1975), Kübler-Ross (1975), Levy and Balfour Sclare (1976), Lewis (1961), Parkes (1964 and 1972), Pincus (1976), Rees & Lutkins (1967), Schmale, Torrie (1970), Weiner.

The Education of Attitudes to Death and Bereavement

Much of the work of this study group was concerned with exposing (and hopefully, educating) the attitudes of mature, experienced and case-hardened professionals. Not surprisingly, this exercise was time-consuming: to translate the experience into syllabuses and procedures for in-service training would be to propose extensive and demanding routines. A panoply of methods would be required: 'non-directed' groups; video-tape, film and role-play case studies; well-prepared inter-professional discussions; deliberately created opportunities to review theory after experience; and the like. Emotional reactions have to be elicited and absorbed. Although the study group seemed convinced that the time and effort would be worthwhile, and the whole exercise 'cost-effective', no-one underestimated the scale of the enterprise.

What, then, of the education of the *general public* in these matters? On the one hand, they are largely ignorant of the issues, so there is much preliminary work to be done; but on the other hand, they are not bound by institutionalised professional practices, and so are able to approach these matters without preconceptions. Might not the task of educating the public be easier? I fear not. Much talk about 'public education' seems to assume that members of the public are not only ignorant but have *no predisposition at all*: simply to inform them of the facts would be to determine their attitudes. Alas, it is not so easy. Especially on such private and value-laden issues as death and grief, the public already have only too deeply entrenched attitudes and emotional predispositions: and these, too, are firmly institutionalised, closely interwoven with the fabric of daily living. True, the form of institutionalisation is *different*, but the pain of self-awareness and change is as searing. And, whereas professionals have some *motive* for educating themselves in such matters, the lay public rarely find themselves in a position which makes such demands. Trapped by social conventions, institutionalised attitudes and emotions, and lack of any motivation, the general public offer an even greater educational challenge. Despite the undoubted quality of many BBC 'Horizon' and 'Man Alive' programmes, Citizen's Advice Bureau pamphlets and the like, the lasting *effects* can hardly be measured.

As I see it, progress in these matters—both in the education of professionals and of the lay public—must go hand in hand with *institutional change*. Increasing the flow of information is certainly necessary, but it is not sufficient: attitudes are bound by social structures—adjustment to new information is normally minimal. With the professions, a re-examination of educational aims, in *all* aspects of the syllabus, is called for. But even this is insufficient, for it raises questions about the aims and social position of the professions themselves—and these questions have a wide relevance to society as a whole. But people, in general, have great difficulty in thinking about their social institutions, the effects of those institutions upon them, and possible changes in those institutions. To enable doctors and nurses to come to terms with their own emotions and attitudes, realistically and creatively, is one thing—and difficult enough in all conscience; but to assist people to find ways by which they can examine, assimilate, learn and *remould* the effect of our social institutions on their attitudes and values—professional or lay—is quite another, and even more difficult, matter. Essentially, the latter problem is one of finding an appropriate *language* to do justice to our experience, and to allow us rationally to reshape it.

To my mind, the education of professional attitudes and values is only worthwhile if it is linked to, and is a catalyst for, institutional change. For education, this implies two key points: i) a much greater emphasis on an appropriate *style* of education, and ii) a greater awareness of the sociological factors which help determine attitudes. Our task is to create an ('artificial', 'structured') environment in which people can display their emotions, and learn an appropriate language in which to discuss and reflect upon their experience. Simulation games, for instance, are *not* child's play; they have to be understood, and seen to be essential, in relation to the development of informed professional self-understanding. In my experience, sociology can provide the appropriate language: science students often find that a sociological understanding makes fresh sense of their own experience, and of many otherwise puzzling features of science and of its public roles and functions. In particular, the sociology of science and of scientific knowledge can now offer convincing explanations of the evolution and tenacity of certain values and practices in the scientific community.[1] Similarly, doctors

[1] I argue the case for a sociological component in scientific training in my paper on 'Moral Education and the Study of Science', in G. Collier, J. Wilson

and nurses should be introduced to a sociological understanding of how values become institutionalised — of how, for instance, values can be a product of a particular process of training—or of the social roots and implications of the claim often advanced by doctors that, 'of course, the decisions involved in terminal care of the dying are purely technical matters—no ethical dilemmas arise in practice, I can assure you.' Unless professionals can imaginatively detach themselves, in appropriate language, from the process of their socialisation, and the structures which perpetuate its effects, they will not be able to reflect critically upon it.

When these points were discussed by the group, it was emphasised that we must attack the problems of professional education with a *variety* of methods. The following practical measures were mentioned as examples of what might be done: whether they amount to 'institutional change' I leave to the reader to judge; —

(a) *Interpersonal sensitivity training*: This should be introduced early in professional training, as soon as it becomes acceptable to examine motives and attitudes critically. Programmes must be carried out professionally to command the respect of students and senior teachers. There should be provision for proper objective assessment, as well as encouragement for self-assessment, and for more open and varied types of assessment.

(b) *Developing capacities for professional self-criticism*: Sociology and the behavioural sciences should be introduced in such a way that they are related more directly to the needs of professional training, with an emphasis on developing professional self-insight, and providing trainees with a language in which to talk and reflect about their own and institutional values.

(c) *Peer-group review and education*: There should be more provision in training for peer-group based review of theory after experience, and opportunities for de-briefing after traumatic experience. There should also be more provision for peer-review and in-service training for qualified professionals.

(d) *Inter-professional contact*: Both in professional education

---

and P. Tomlinson (eds), *Values and Moral Development in Higher Education* (London: Croom Helm, 1974), pp. 147–59. For a particular example of sociological explication of values and their functions, see M. J. Mulkay, 'Norms and Ideology in Science', *Social Science Information*, Vol. 15 (1976), pp. 637–56. For further readings and references, see B. Barnes (ed.), *Sociology of Science* (Harmondsworth, Middx.: Penguin Modern Sociology Readings, 1972), and I. Spiegel-Rösing and D. de S. Price (eds), *Science, Technology and Society: A Cross-Disciplinary Perspective* (London and Beverly Hills, Calif.: SAGE Publications, 1977).

and professional practice there should be provision for inter-professional training—cspecially in areas like terminal care, where team co-operation is essential.

(e) *Apprenticeship*: In teaching the art of medicine anyone with the appropriate skill and insight can be a teacher, and the 'elders of the tribe' have a particularly significant contribution to make. Proper supervision and de-briefing of trainees can be the most valuable form of training—especially in relation to Death and Bereavement—but it needs to be more formally incorporated in to medical and professional training.

David Edge

Appendixes

Appendix 1

Recommendations Relating to Professional Training and
Involvement in the Care of the Dying and the Bereaved

IN ADDITION TO the regular meetings of the Working Group special meetings
were convened of professional sub-groups representing each of the following—
Doctors, Nurses, Social Workers and Ministers. Special efforts were made to
ensure that these groups were as fully representative as possible of the professions concerned. The purpose of convening these groups was to test out the
validity of some of the conclusions reached in the larger multi-disciplinary
Working Group, and to formulate policy statements regarding the appropriate
involvement of Doctors, Nurses, Social Workers and Ministers in the care of
the dying and the bereaved.

Medical Viewpoint

It was generally agreed that it is easier to recognise the good than to define the
ideal in relation to the care of the dying and the bereaved. The group were most
concerned with practical measures to improve standards of care and no ideal
check-list of specific obligations to the dying and the bereaved was produced.
It was recognised that in 'real-life' medicine there was room for improvement.
There was extended discussion of the difficulties faced by hospital and family
doctors, and of the various limitations of time and facilities which contribute
to standards of care in some instances being less than desirable. Serious defects
were noted in the current training of medical students in this area—both with
respect to their attitudes towards the care of the dying and the bereaved and in
the techniques of good terminal care. The neglect or evasion of the topics of
death and bereavement in the medical curriculum was deplored.

The main emphasis in the group was on the need for an adequate standard of
technical competence among doctors in the management of pain and other
symptoms in the dying patient. Although it was felt that the broad principles
of the therapeutics of terminal care are known in the profession, it was regretted
that most doctors remain in ignorance of the details of the growing literature
in the field.

In relation to medical attitudes to death it was agreed that in cure-orientated
medicine death tends to be seen as a failure and professional set-back for the
doctor. The negative attitude was implicated as a factor in the mismanagement
of certain categories of patient and as encouraging doctors to over-investigate
patients in the course of 'striving officiously to keep alive'. Many senior doctors,
and most geriatricians, saw death in certain circumstances as appropriate,
timely and acceptable to the patient and professionals alike. Age, the nature
of the disease process and the previous quality of life contributed to the assessment of the death as 'not premature'. A secular change in public attitudes to
death, in step with changing epidemiological patterns, was noted: 'young' death
was now rarer, 'old' death commoner in the community than formerly.

170

Much attention was given to the problems of communicating with and around the dying patient. It was agreed that the truth should be told 'as much as was consistent with good patient care'. The concept of communication by silence, not necessarily evasive, and the 'positiveness of doing nothing' were both noted. The idea of seeking identification with the dying patient as an optional basis for communicating with him was discussed at some length, and met with general approval. This process was both demanding and time-consuming, and was very much the ideal rather than the average standard of practice. The great variation in communication skills between different members of the profession was noted. It was agreed that in this area more than any other, there was both room for, and hope of, improvement. Individuals might exist who, even with appropriate training, might never learn to communicate adequately, though others might, as a result of their own sensitivity or fortunate experience in the observation of their senior mentors, perform well without any specific instruction. The idea that medical students should be screened in some way for such skills before commencing the course was discarded, as the predictive value of such an exercise was questionable. There was emphatic support for the idea that general standards could be improved by the promotion of a fairly simple set of 'do's' and 'don'ts' to be inculcated at the undergraduate level. There is a distinction to be drawn between doctors having different levels of skill in the care of the dying, and no awareness at all. 'If it is possible to think about what's wrong with medical practice then it is possible to think how it could be improved, and then skills can be developed and training methods devised.'

One of the chief problems in the care of the dying, with particular bearing on the bereavement of the patient and which creates complications for the relatives, is the difficulty of maintaining continuity of care by the same staff. However, it was felt that it was virtually impossible to do anything about it in the present set-up in general hospitals and only the creation of special terminal care units could possibly meet this need.

There was less convergence of thinking on the question of the care, if necessary, of the bereaved; bereavement was not generally accepted as 'a temporary psychological illness'. Some doctors (of the 'Life is tough' school) considered it is an unavoidable part of full human experience. In general the value of a surveillance remit, with follow-up after an interval, at which lingering questions might be discussed, was recognised; but the dangers of the medicalisation of bereavement were noted. The place of lay people—whether relatives, neighbours, volunteers or non-medical professionals—in the care/surveillance of the bereaved, was recognised and the doctor's responsibility to co-operate with and encourage this assistance was emphasised. Community contributions were held to be of most value in normal bereavement, but the duty of recognising pathological grief reactions was agreed to fall within the province certainly of the medical and possibly of the nursing profession.

Training of medical students in terminal care
AIMS
   A. Creating an awareness of the following:
   1. The practical problems for patients and family.
   2. The emotional problems for patients and family.
   3. The practical problems for nurses.
   4. The emotional problems for nurses and colleagues.
   5. The need for a long-term view, particularly in preparation for bereavement of relatives.
   6. The need for a co-ordinated, team approach to the whole problem from the time when it becomes apparent that no further curative measures apply.

B. Developing an *understanding* of:
1. The need for a *positive* policy which can bring all manner of practical and emotional support into action *if and when* it is needed without needless interference or medical meddling with what can often be regarded as a sad but physiological fact.
2. The emotional burden on relatives, starting as it does even before the patient may be aware that an illness is terminal, lasting throughout the final phases of the illness, and on through bereavement, that the relatives may have dreaded but never spoken of to anyone.
3. The difficulties of communication with all concerned, patients, relatives, colleagues of all disciplines, and the need for a sensitive awareness of the problems at each stage, even before the 'terminal' phase has started clinically.

By *example*, to try to develop a truly *sympathetic* yet positive attitude to death and its problems.

METHODS

The material cannot all be taught in the same ordered, scientific manner as most other clinical problems. Some or all of the following methods might be employed:

1. Teaching of this subject should take place somewhere about the middle of their clinical course. If it is placed too early it will appear theoretical and insufficiently attached to clinical cases. If it appears too late it will be rejected as non-examination material.

2. Advice should be obtained from specialists on the management of dying in specific situations, e.g. in intensive care units and in paediatric hospitals.

3. The subject should be included in teaching programmes when students are attached to general practices.

4. Tutorials, with the involvement of a patient or relatives, if they are willing to do so, perhaps in the new St Columba's Hospice, and in conjunction with the domiciliary care which will be operated from St Columba's Hospice. Within hospital the material should be heavily case-orientated, either in the form of case summaries, or around specific patients dying in the ward. Thus, opportunities will be provided to see patients and relatives at home, in hospitals and in the new Hospice and to observe team work which is desirable in the management of patient and relatives.

5. Tutorials should be run for doctors and nurses together, as, in this way, the fact that the problem is, at present at least, one for medical and nursing staff will be emphasised. Tutor groups should be set up involving a general practitioner, a hospital doctor, a nurse and an appropriately experienced member of another profession, e.g. the ministry or social work.

6. Short-term attachment, either as resident student or nursing auxiliary to the Hospice.

We believe that benefits will be obtained from students receiving guidance alongside nurses, social workers and other paramedical professions, but also including theological students. These methods are not yet used to any real extent in our present teaching hospitals where the benefits of mutual co-operation and interdependence are only slowly being realised.

MATERIALS

A. *Death:* Death as a physiological phenomenon, its signs and symptoms, the increasing difficulty in discerning and ascertaining death due to support machinery—distinction between somatic and cerebral death—the element of urgency involved in the need for transplant surgery accepted by the community.

The concept of premature death and of timely death—distinguishing between less common premature death in youth and much more common timely death in age. Differences in management.

B. *Dying:* Idea of pre-death, mainly, but not entirely geriatric, i.e. a totally dependent state short of death. Difficulty of deciding when is 'dying'. Distinction between living with a mortal disease and actually dying which is a shorter experience. Psychological changes involved in dying, loneliness, fear, anger, acceptance. Considerable emphasis on fear which involves all patients and includes fear of pain, loss of personal happiness, loss of family, fear of the unknown, fear of institutions, fear of 'hell'. Death not feared, but rather the accompaniments of dying, e.g. pain, nausea, dyspnoea, fatigue, loss of physiological function, loss of dignity, loss of mental stability. Need for increased, rather than decreased, doctor involvement in the care of the dying. Need for close attention to relief of symptoms. St Christopher drug list. Drugs not a substitute for personal contact.

C. *General management of all patients, including the dying:* Balance of acceptable and unacceptable experiences leading to acceptance of death. Too great a pathological load leading to a desire for death. Wishes of patients in this respect are not self-pitying but truthful and accurate assessments of the situation, therefore non-specific untrue assurances of health by medical staff are cruel and inefficient. Settling for comfort once terminal phase is clear. Decision by the consensus. Limited consultation with relatives and patient. Need for clear idea of doctors' aims and goals for patient. Avoidance of treatment merely to satisfy doctor, relatives or other staff. 'Settling for comfort and relief of distress'—not merely stopping drips, injections, resuscitations, etc., but initiation of a positive regime with different goals. Difficult decisions in case of bleeding patients, patients developing gangrene, etc., where surgery may be difficult to reject. Need for relief of distress, using whatever drugs and whatever doses are required to achieve this. Irrelevance of drug addiction in terminal phase. Some patients live with very limited lives which may be unacceptable to medical attendant. Medical attendants' assessment of value patient places on life is irrelevant if patient available for consultation. Difficulties arising where patient not available for consultation, e.g. severe dementia, coma, etc. No investigation without possibility of treatment. Emphasis on continuity of management between hospital and general practice if patient moving between these. Usual poor hospital/general practice contact doubly unacceptable in the care of the dying.

D. *Should the doctor tell?:* Repeated short discussions with patient. Patient must be allowed to converse. Interviews should not merely be the giving of information. Need for frankness and avoidance of lies and deceit. Tell the patient if he asks, but afford him the opportunity to ask. Answer only the question which is asked. Don't say more than you know about prognosis. If the patient asks, it is because he wants to know for better or for worse. Eighty per cent of patients dying know that they are dying. Influence of relatives on telling the patient. Firm statement that if the patient asks he must be told, no matter what the relatives may wish. Who should tell? Generally the most senior person, not doctors or nurses in training. Need for empathic person more important than seniority or experience. Use of appropriate terminology, avoidance of scare words, e.g. cancer. Accept patient's religious beliefs and expressions without denial or ridicule. Make clear whether we are communicating the disease label, no time scale mentioned, or merely the time scale, or both. Cancer should be cut down to size, i.e. only one of many mortal diseases, by public education. Within that context patients and relatives have opportunity to change lifestyle for final phase of life, or, conversely, may have final phase of life blighted by cloud of impending doom. This problem only solved by close, continuous and sympathetic contact. Communicating 'I don't know'; many patients tolerate uncertainty, many patients have anxiety for the doctor and his feelings.

E. *Management of relatives:* As above. Frankness, avoidance of conspiracy, implying cessation of common practice of telling a close relative but not the patient of a serious prognosis. Persuade relatives that truth is best. Advise relatives of possibility of death in advance, if possible. Offer the opportunity for home care and avoidance of hospital admission by frank acceptance of fact that patient is dying.

F. *General interview technique.* Applicable in all situations.

(a) Sitting, not across the table, but close to patients; (b) give impressions that time is no object, i.e. by not standing up, looking at watch, etc.; (c) let patient talk for short period; (d) some interviews should be totally private, with not even a nurse present; (e) get facts concerning patient up to date before sitting down with patient, avoid rifling through notes before patient; (f) instruction on use of touch, eye-to-eye contact; (g) no laughter which does not include patient, i.e. not between staff members at bed end; (h) avoid head-shaking under all circumstances; (i) avoid sinister examination of X-rays before patient; (j) avoid technical discussions across patient unless patient included; (k) barriers between patient and doctor—i. knowledge and education, ii. class, iii. age, iv. sex, v. fear of patient, vi. well doctor versus unwell patient, vii. 'panoply of profession', viii. old charity basis of medicine lives on, especially in the hospitals, (l) use proper title—'Mrs, Miss, Mrs' not 'gran', 'pop', 'dear', 'ducks'; (m) don't ignore patients to converse with students, nurses, etc.; (n) don't let silence develop in interviews; (o) deal gently but firmly with tears but don't terminate interview; (p) no swearing, mateyness and other patronising behaviour; (q) don't exhibit anger in the clinical situation, retire to office if necessary; (r) don't criticise other doctors or staff in the patient's presence.

Under the heading of general interview technique the students should be instructed in the structure of a general interview, i.e. introduction, general conversation, passive phase of interview, inquisition phase of interview and final information in what will follow in the patient's management. There are several good small textbooks available on interview technique. Each of the above headings is capable of considerable expansion, depending on the experience and capabilities of the tutors.

Nurses' Viewpoint

The nurses' sub-group discussed nursing involvement with the dying and the bereaved and formulated an explicit list of nursing values applicable to nursing responsibilities in this area:

1. To value care of the dying and the bereaved as a positive, important and skilled function of nurses. 2. To appreciate the importance of providing care for both the dying person and the significant other(s); and of providing continuity of care throughout the phases of pre-death, death and bereavement. 3. To contribute to the overall assessment of the needs of the dying person and the significant other(s); and to assist in co-ordinating the support and services of appropriate professions. 4. To ensure that the care provided to the dying and the bereaved accommodates their choices and wishes wherever possible, so that the individual's dignity and autonomy is preserved during this unique life experience. 5. To provide a major contribution towards ensuring the dying person's maximum physical comfort in relation to basic physical needs on the basis of a nursing assessment. 6. To make a major contribution in providing emotional and psychological support to the dying person and the bereaved on the basis of personal involvement, compassion and knowledge of the emotional experiences met in the processes of dying and bereavement. 7. To respect the spiritual beliefs

and needs of the dying person (whatever the nurse's own beliefs may be). 8. To allow the significant other(s) to become involved (or not) in the care and support of the dying person; and to prepare them for bereavement and provide appropriate help and support. 9. To assist the doctor in providing medical care, at the same time protecting the dying patient from inappropriate medical investigation or treatment. 10. To attempt to communicate the event of death to the significant other(s) in the least distressing way. 11. To assume a responsibility towards educating and supporting nursing colleagues and students in the care of the dying and the bereaved. 12. To ascept a responsibility to develop nursing knowledge and skills in the care of the dying and the bereaved.

The recommendations of the Nurses' sub-group on the training and involvement of nurses in the care of the dying and the bereaved are set out in the following:—

Care of the dying in hospital: This is a function of all hospital nurses and a major function of some (e.g. medical, intensive care, geriatric nursing). It involves deaths in all age groups and 'sudden' as well as 'slow degenerative' deaths. Nursing care varies according to the patient's age, disease condition, length of pre-death phase, family and social circumstances, degree of dependence, awareness of approaching death, emotional reactions, religion and spiritual needs, and choices and wishes about his care. Nursing includes physical care, administration of medically-prescribed treatments, and emotional support. Hospital nurses have limited contact with the patient's family. 'Individualised' care is desirable, but difficult.

The major problems include fragmentation of care (due to shifts and 'job allocation' system); communication problems (with patient, relatives, other staff); conflicting values of caring for the 'ill' and carying for the dying; the lack of privacy in hospital wards; the young age of student nurses and the inexperience of untrained 'nurses' (together making up the largest proportion of nursing manpower).

2. *Caring for the dying at home:* This is an important function of the District Nurse. Her role differs in that care is provided on an intermittent but individual basis; she works in close contact with the patient's family; she acts as an independent practitioner; she works with a limited number of other professionals with whom she has regular contact (e.g. the GP). Nursing care involves physical care for the patient, emotional support of patient and family, and practical help and guidance for the family. The DN has the advantage of being older and, qualified as a nurse, has experience of care of the dying.

The main problems include practical difficulties of the environment; reconciling the needs and wishes of the patient and the family (that may be in conflict); and ensuring that appropriate help is forthcoming from other professionals.

Care of the bereaved: Nurses have a less obvious role, but contribution includes:—1. preparation for bereavement of the dying patient's family during the pre-death phase (hospital and community); 2. the brief, but significant, encounter (in the hospital setting) with the bereaved immediately post-death (sometimes to communicate the event, usually to deal with practicalities of the deceased person's effects); 3. in hospital, nursing recently bereaved patients (e.g. survivor of a multiple accident, elderly bereaved spouse admitted for social reasons, perinatal death); 4. in community DN may provide informal support for the family of a patient she nursed (although this is not a statutory function) and DN or HV may be involved incidentally with patients or clients who are bereaved.

General responsibilities towards the dying and bereaved: include:—1. an educational role in improving public's understanding of death and bereavement; 2. a professional role in improving nursing knowledge and education related; 3. a 'political' role in pressing for improvements in provisions for care of the dying and the bereaved.

Education of nurses in the care of the dying and the bereaved

Any practical recommendations about education must be considered in the context: the contribution nurses make to the care of the dying and bereaved; problems experienced in the provision of this care; the limitations inherent in the present educational system.

In other words, aims of education need to be relevant to nursing practice and goals must be attainable within the limitations of the present system of nurse training. Some of these limitations are outlined below:

(a) The student nurse is an employee first and a student second—and so planned, sequential and standardised teaching is seldom possible.

(b) The student nurse starts nursing right from the start of training. Although it is sometimes useful to teach on the basis of some first-hand experience of the subject, death is less suitable for this approach because of the young age of student nurses ($17\frac{1}{2}$ years upwards).

(c) Nurse training (i.e. a standard 3-year training for registration) is divided into 'clinical experience' (about 100 weeks) and 'classroom teaching' (about 30 weeks). These two components do not relate in time and so integration of theory and practice is difficult. The learning experience is further fragmented by different people teaching in these components (tutors in the classroom and clinical staff in the wards). For the students this tends to polarise 'the theoretical' and 'the practical'. For the staff it means that teaching staff may be out of touch with the reality; and clinical staff may be out-of-date in terms of knowledge and content of classroom teaching.

(d) Being basically an apprenticeship system, nurse training relies on the student nurse learning while working. There are obvious advantages, but many limitations that are not fully appreciated. For example, students now move about from speciality to speciality more frequently and spend less time on the wards and so their clinical experience is fragmented: it is seldom possible to provide a logical sequence of experience for an individual student nurse; within any student group the experiences will vary widely and so make classroom teaching difficult. The assumption that student nurses are apprentices and learn from the example of senior colleagues fails to take account of the reality—that students more often work alone or with each other or with an untrained 'nurse' than with a trained member of staff and, when available, ward nurses often fail to exploit the students' clinical experience as a learning opportunity.

Different aims would need to be identified for different nurses' training programmes to take account of the type and degree of involvement in death and bereavement that such trained nurses would have. Some programmes would have limited aims (e.g. psychiatric nurse training) and others would require a large component (e.g. DN training, courses in geriatric nursing such as the JBCNS post-basic course). For the purpose of this exercise, practical recommendations are made for basic *general* nurse training (i.e. 3-year course leading to RGN). Teaching and learning about death and bereavement could aim to:—

1. Promote understanding of the contribution, values and goals of the nursing profession in the care of the dying and the bereaved.

2. Develop understanding, and application to practice, of knowledge about the processes and problems of death and bereavement.

3. Promote competence in:
   nursing assessment of dying patients, their families and bereaved people,

the provisions of physical nursing care for dying patients, meeting the emotional needs of dying patients, their families and bereaved people.

4. Create an awareness of personal feelings about death and develop appropriate ways of coping personally with the emotional demands of professional care for the dying and the bereaved.

5. Clarify the roles in the care of the dying and bereaved of other professionals and involved groups; identify areas of conflict and difficulty; and promote a constructive approach to teamwork.

Practical recommendations for education of nurses in the care of the dying and the bereaved

Working from the aims identified, education could be attempted by a 'teaching' component provided within classroom teaching and a 'learning' component based on clinical experience. The aims identified intend to stress the importance of nurses obtaining a general understanding of death and bereavement, as well as a personal one, as a background to learning about the practicalities of nursing care for the dying and the bereaved.

Classroom teaching would best be coped with as a specific course on 'death and bereavement' during one of the early blocks (perhaps during the second half of the first year). Timed then, the students would have some experience to relate to teaching but it would not be too late to be of use during the main part of training.

The course could include the following topics:—epidemiological facts of death; sociological aspects of death and bereavement; death as a physiological phenomenon; medical diagnosis of death (including difficulties of time prognosis); types of death (sudden, timely, premature); features of the pre-death phase; physical problems associated with dying and related nursing care; psychological and emotional problems associated with dying, and related nursing care; pain control in terminal illness; concept of death as loss; reactions to death (grief, shock, disbelief, denial, awareness, acceptance, etc.); the practical and emotional problems of the illness, knowledge of prognosis, pre-death and death for the dying patient's family (*N.B.* identification of the significant others); the processes and problems of bereavement (anticipatory grieving; short- and long-term features of bereavement; social attitudes and customs; absent, delayed or inhibited grief; depression, hypochondriasis and illness; medicalisation of bereavement); advantages and disadvantages of hospital and home deaths; roles of health-care professionals and other groups (e.g. clergy, police, undertakers, CRUSE); the team approach to care; inter-professional conflicts and moral dilemmas; specific contribution, values and goals of the nursing profession; communicating with dying patients, their relatives and other professionals; the relationship between nurses, the patient and his family (the difficulties, defence mechanisms).

The list of topics seems very long and the time available would dictate how deeply the topics could be broached. However, a superficial coverage of the breadth of the subject of death and bereavement would seem better than a narrow concentration on nursing procedures and the important aspects related to nursing care can be taught and learned in the clinical areas.

A combination of teaching methods could be used—lectures, talks by other professionals, documentary films, informal discussion groups, case-based discussions and reading.

The specific course could be backed up and extended in other teaching courses and additional material included in relevant other courses (e.g. child death in paediatrics).

Clinical teaching and learning by experience must be considered as complimentary to the classroom courses and must be as well planned. Clinical teachers, ward staff and tutors (who do venture into the wards) would need to be encouraged to consider dying patients as 'teaching material' as valuable as ill patients or patients requiring technical nursing care. A planned teaching session with a dying patient would help a student nurse to apply her knowledge, practise assessment, implement physical care, and provide emotional support with the teacher's guidance and help and example. In discussion, after the session, the student could be encouraged to discuss the patient as a dying patient and to express her anxieties about this kind of nursing role. Such planned clinical teaching sessions are increasingly provided for student nurses and the dying patient is just another category of patient that should be included in teaching of this nature.

Ward nursing staff could be encouraged by such example to be more explicit in their supervision of students' work with dying patients and in using the work as a learning experience. Where possible, student nurses should be involved as non-participant observers in nursing contacts with relatives or in joint medical-nursing discussions so that they learn nursing functions usually performed by senior staff.

The nursing report and informal ward tutorials both provide ideal opportunities for discussion of nursing care of the dying as a learning situation for student nurses.

Making more explicit the clinical teaching component of education about death and bereavement could also be aided by ensuring that student nurses do gain experience in practice of caring for dying patients and this could be planned at ward level as well as curriculum level (e.g. an allocation to a geriatric unit).

Interdisciplinary teaching has not been mentioned to date, but some attempt should be made to plan for this in this subject. Many of the interdisciplinary conflicts highlighted in the Working Group arose because education for each profession is so separate and students do not mix during training. Joint education would not remove the conflicts that arise because of different professional ethos and values, but might help to promote an understanding that conflicts exist and that they can only be resolved by mutual discussion and better attempts to implement a team approach.

Because of the different systems of education joint formal teaching is unlikely to be possible. However, an ideal opportunity for this subject would be to hold joint nursing and medical ward tutorials for the discussion of patients in the ward. Second- and third-year nursing students could join tutorials with fourth- or fifth-year medical students and these could be run by members of the nursing and medical staff jointly.

Practical recommendations to encourage improvements in nursing care
Recommendations can only be general and many suggested may operate only in some situations. However, this aspect of nursing practice in general merits scrutiny and on the whole deserves improvement. The comments pertain to hospital care by and large.

1. *Deployment of staff.* Care of the dying is often delegated to inexperienced staff. This implies that it is not skilled and has low status. It also implicitly denies the stress inherent in this role. Where possible, trained and experienced staff should be available to supervise and give emotional support to nurses caring for the dying.

The system of 'job allocation' employed in nursing is as unsuitable for dying patients as for acutely ill patients. Attempts should be made to provide a system of individualised care. This is even more demanding for the nurses involved and so selection of staff becomes even more important. It should be recognised that some nurses may not enjoy or be good at this nursing function.

2. *Communication amongst nurses.* Formal communication—reports and the Kardex—tends to cease to include details when a patient is dying rather than ill, and reduces to verbal comments such as 'I see he's still with us this morning' and written comments such as 'total nursing care'. These sorts of instructions are useless and nurses need to be fully informed about medical treatment, prognosis, physical requirements, emotional state, communications to patient and relatives. The ward sister (or nurse in charge) must assume the responsibility to ensure full verbal reports and written instructions and stress the importance of communication of observations made about the patient by the nurses. Improved nursing communication will mean that nurses are better informed and, as a result, will have confidence to relate to the patient and will give appropriate care.

3. *Communication between nurses and doctors.* Of crucial importance is that doctors give full details of 'medical information' to nurses and nurses do likewise with 'nursing information'. The nursing staff need to know from the medical staff (a) the prognosis and changes in medical condition; (b) decisions about resuscitation or not and; (c) *exactly* what the doctor has told the patient and relatives about the prognosis and what he has learned from them that might be relevant to nursing. Without this information nurses cannot care effectively for dying patients and, to avoid difficult questions, adopt defence mechanisms (such as avoidance of the patient and visitors; referral of questions to others; over-emphasis on physical nursing; denial of prognosis; hoping for a miracle cure; or adopting a cheerful or cool composure). All this prohibits the patient from expressing his fears, worries and wishes and he senses alienation and loses trust in the nurses. It is the doctor's responsibility to ensure that nurses have this information and nurses' understanding of the implications of specific diagnoses should not be overestimated. Equally, nurses have a responsibility to communicate their observations to the medical staff (e.g. about the patient's pain control).

The obvious line of doctor-nurse communication is the ward sister but as she is there for 38 hours only, communication must be made to the nurse in charge. Discussion and joint planning should be attempted in addition to this to-and-fro exchange of information.

4. *Communication between nurses and dying patients/emotional support* would be greatly improved if, (a) nurses were better educated about death and dying; (b) were better informed about the patient and; (c) if emotional support was provided for them. The prognosis of death seems to put a barrier between patients and nurses and when truthfulness is not the policy (or when nurses don't know who has been told what) then the only approach is the conspiracy of silence and the adoption of defence mechanisms. It may also be true that nurses are taught to 'cope' and 'not get involved' and so emotional situations are avoided in order to avoid their consequences. Effective communication is the basis of providing emotional support and so is crucial to the total care of the patient. If nurses are aware of their own and the patient's reactions to death, then they should be able to more realistically approach the task of using communication in assisting the patient to cope with his approaching death. The fear that nurses will be faced with the direct question 'Am I dying?' is largely unfounded and the elaborate avoidance of the possibility of this question arising puts limitations on any interaction. Anyway, if the patient asks he wants to know; and, if the nurse knows the prognosis, she can then cope with the question.

Listening to the patient is far more important than talking to him, and by

179

listening the nurses will gain an understanding of his needs and worries. Cheerfulness and coolness, often useful in nursing, are probably inappropriate and involvement and expression of sympathy and compassion should be encouraged —TLC in the best sense of the term. This can be achieved from a personal rather than professional approach and possible if the nurse can cope with her own feelings and reactions. Spending time with the patient, being patient over physical care, listening, being close (by touch and eye contact), keeping silent if appropriate, and spontaneous conversation are ways to show compassion, alleviate the feeling of loneliness in dying, and assist the patient in coming to terms with his death. All this is difficult to teach because it seems 'soft' but it seems to have got lost in the stress on clinical competence in nursing.

5. *Communication between nurses and relatives/significant others* would improve if nurses were informed about their patients and had closer relationships with the dying patient. Effective communication with relatives is an important medium in preparation for bereavement and in assisting them to come to terms with the approaching death. Avoidance of relatives is widely practised and deliberate attempts should be made to let visitors know that nurses are available to talk and give information. The 'busy' front is used to fend off relatives of all kinds of patients but, when the patient is dying, this is not permissible. The ward is the relative's only contact with the person about to die and every opportunity should be made to allow them privacy, choice and involvement. Nurses can seem much more approachable than doctors who relatives often perceive as too busy, distant or important, to bother with trivial questions. The nurse can ask the doctor to see the relatives or can interpret medical information as well as discuss the fears and anxieties the relatives may have. Practical advice about visiting may be helpful or necessary. Allowing relatives to be involved in the actual care of the patient (e.g. feeding, washing, etc.) can give them a purpose to visit, and allow expression of concern and love. All this may mean that nursing routine may have to be relaxed or altered and a degree of privacy allowed. Again nurses should be encouraged to communicate on a personal rather than professional level.

Prior discussion and decision on practical matters can greatly alleviate difficulties later—e.g. do relatives want to be telephoned at night? The decision can then be noted in the Kardex.

The immediate post-death contact is highly significant as it is the first explicit confirmation of the death. Nurses should be prepared for a variety of reactions —shock, grief, disbelief, denial, anger—and deal with these kindly. Genuine kindness and dealing with practicalities (e.g. how is she going to get home?) are probably much more helpful than the regulation cup of tea.

Requests to see the body should always be allowed (those who will find it disturbing won't ask).

Giving the deceased person's effects to the relatives at this point is a crucial procedure and some alternative should be sought (e.g. a central office at which collection could be made later).

6. *Physical nursing care of the dying* is probably least in need of improvement, although better knowledge about the physical changes and problems would help nurses to provide appropriate care. Care includes—nursing measures to alleviate pain, anorexia or nausea, dehydration, discomforts of the mouth, dyspnoea, sleep problems, temperature regulation problems, constipation, odours, etc. and to compensate for loss of independence in mobility, elimination functions, failing vision and hearing and general weakness. Dying patients seem to become much more sensitive to 'minor' discomforts such as pressure from bedclothes, light and noise, and so tremendous patience and skill are needed to help the patient to be comfortable. For a fully conscious patient, loss

of independence in basic activities of daily living is difficult to accept and nurses should not enforce helplessness upon a patient able and wishing to help to look after his basic needs. Tact and sympathy can help to minimise the loss of self-respect and the indignity of dying. Changes in physical appearance can be distressing and morale can be improved by careful grooming.

In the late stages nursing pride in cleanliness, order and routine must be sacrificed to the benefit of the patient's comfort and wishes. Overzealous physical nursing (e.g. prevention of pressure sores) should be prevented. The patient's peace, dignity and comfort are the priorities.

There can be tremendous satisfaction for nurses in caring well for a dying patient and good physical care can be an important expression of care, concern and respect for the person. Lack of time and conflicting priorities in the ward can result in dissatisfaction and nurses may feel guilty and distressed that good care was not given to the patient.

7. *Ward management.* Caring for dying patients is in conflict with a ward routine designed to care for the ill, but alive. Time and privacy are needed if good care is to be given and a system of individual total care makes different demands than the usual 'job allocation' system. Adaptations to the routine are needed and the needs of the dying must be considered to be important, even if the needs of the living must sometimes take priority.

Privacy for the patient and his visitors is difficult to secure in an open ward but a single room may be available (if this is in the interests of all concerned) or the patient's bed could be moved to a quiet part of the ward. Moving beds around is often not helpful to anyone and it may just be better to make good use of bed screens for privacy.

The conspiracy to exclude all other patients from a death in the ward demands elaborate rituals and untruthfulness and is probably unhelpful to those it is meant to protect. It is a delicate problem, but one that nurses should think about more carefully. Awareness of the emotional reactions of other patients is crucial and their needs (other than unhealthy curiosity) should be met by discussion and explanation. In long-stay wards (e.g. geriatrics) some patients may be bereaved from a death in the ward and require support. The practice of screening all beds for the removal of a body is probably quite unnecessary and if the procedure was done openly, but discreetly, it would permit acknowledgment of the event and thus allow the members of the ward (staff and patients) to express reactions about the loss.

This procedure is indicative of the quick 'clearing-up' operation that follows a death in the ward and, in general, post-death management need not be rushed in this way. For nurses, a death in their off-duty is communicated by a gap in the Kardex and an empty bed and it would be much more helpful for the information to be explicitly communicated, for example by a brief 'post-mortem' report

Ministers' Viewpoint
Ministry to the dying and the bereaved
The main issues discussed were: (a) the conduct of funerals and discussion of their significance; (b) the Catholic practice of praying for the dead, its theological basis and pastoral value; (c) the differences between dealing with believers and non-believers; (d) the responsibility of minister and worshipping community to support the bereaved; (e) (*pastoral*) care for the dying; (f) areas of conflict with other professions; (g) recommendations for improved training of clergy.

(a) *The conduct of funerals.* There was marked divergence on the question of the primary purpose and significance of funeral services. The C of S ministers emphasised that the funeral is an occasion for giving spiritual comfort and expressing personal sympathy to the bereaved family and friends of the dead, that it is an occasion for the cathartic expression of grief. The R.C. and Episcopalian ministers stressed the primary significance of the funeral as an act of worship ('holding the dead in the presence of God'), as an act of celebration and prayer for the dead, and that it is only secondarily concerned with comforting and exhorting the congregation. However, it was agreed that there are two foci of a funeral—the dead person in the coffin and the family. There was considerable convergence on the following issues. (i) That a funeral should be an occasion for affirmation of faith, hope and assurance in the grace and mercy of God. (ii) That it should be an occasion for truthful and frank recognition of the fact of death, and encouragement to us to accept our mortality. (iii) That it should be an occasion for both thanksgiving and frank expression of grief and sympathy, including so far as possible truthful acceptance of the real character of the person deceased.

(b) *Prayers for the dead—differing views.* There was frank disagreement on the value of the Catholic practice of masses and prayers for the dead. On the one hand it was questioned whether these did not encourage morbid attitudes, impose added burdens on the bereaved and encourage In-Memoriam type gestures which were concerned more with self-advertisement than genuine thanksgiving or expression of grief. On the other hand the practice was justified on theological and pastoral grounds—as giving concrete expression to the doctrine of the Communion of Saints and as canalising the grief and often contradictory feelings of the bereaved towards the dead and towards themselves. It was also emphasised that memorial masses on monthly and annual anniversaries can be of great comfort to the bereaved at times when they particularly need support.

(c) *Relations with unbelievers.* It was frankly recognised that a large percentage of funerals concern individuals or families with little or no connection with the Church. In this context it was emphasised that there are a number of things the minister should try to do.

(i) Get to know as much as possible about the dead person and his family, their attitudes and relationships so that conduct of the funeral and subsequent pastoral support can be given in terms that are both relevant and meaningful —or where this is impossible the set forms should be adhered to and use made of silence, allowing people to fill in the content for themselves.

(ii) That where possible a minister should be involved who has had some contact with the deceased or the family.

(iii) That all people need to be encouraged to face up to the facts of their mortality and ministers have a large part to play in encouraging more frank attitudes to death and suffering. (E.g. the question was raised whether the unpopularity of discussion of the theology of death is not part of the 'conspiracy of silence' about death, and a contributory factor in declining belief in the resurrection unto eternal life.)

(iv) That in counselling the dying or the bereaved it is important to find out where the person stands himself in relation to Church observance and Christian belief and to recognise that people turn to ministers at times of death as much for their familiarity with death and expertise in knowing what has to be done, as for any explicit religious counselling.

(d) *Care for the bereaved.* There was wide consensus on the point that in relation to his pastoral duties the minister ought to give priority to counselling and support for the bereaved. The following points were emphasised:

(i) That ministers ought to make it their business to get to know more about the stages of normal grief reaction as well as its pathological forms.

(ii) That they should educate their parishioners to a more sympathetic understanding of the needs of the bereaved, and the ordinary as well as extra-ordinary forms which grief can take, including the therapeutic value of visions and communication with the dead.

(iii) That ministers are called to a 'ministry of listening', that they should encourage people to talk out their grief, feelings of anger, guilt, remorse.

(iv) That ministers should activate concerned groups to give support to the bereaved (particularly to young parents who have become isolated by the loss of a child, for example).

(v) That ministers should recognise that the grieving process can go on for a long time and that people may need particular support on anniversaries and similar occasions of painful reminder.

(e) *Ministry to the dying*

(i) That ministers have a responsibility to avoid creating a 'conspiracy of silence' around the dying, that frankness should be encouraged while also emphasising the responsibilities which telling the truth entails—by way of giving support and counselling.

(ii) That when possible people should be encouraged to talk about their views of death, their fears of dying and their related anxieties, but they should also be encouraged to affirm their dignity by making of their death a free act.

(iii) That people must be met where they are. That the deathbed is unlikely to be the appropriate place for theological discussion and what may be needed is simple reassurance. (E.g. 'Yes. You will meet your family again in Heaven' may be the most comforting and intelligible form in which the Communion of the Saints can be expressed around a death-bed.)

(iv) It was emphasised that effective care for the physical and spiritual needs of the dying requires the fullest possible consultation and co-operation between the minister, the patient and relatives, the doctor, nurses and hospital staff. The sharing of relevant information is essential if all are to play their proper part.

(v) It was agreed that in general it is in the best interests of the patient and the relatives if death can occur at home. This avoids painful and sometimes tragic separation and isolation of the dying, makes it possible for the family to share in the experience together, makes it possible for the process of grieving to begin naturally and makes the exercise of a more meaningful spiritual ministry possible—to the dying and their relatives. The lack of privacy, lack of time and opportunity for relaxed conversation or prayer in hospital, makes ministry to the dying difficult.

(vi) The 'conspiracy of silence' around the dying was generally deplored and it was stressed that the patient's right to know should always be respected. It was recognised that most dying patients seem to know that they are dying and are generally reassured to know the truth. Conversely, uncertainty about their condition or prognosis were recognised to be the causes of the greatest anxiety in the dying. It was stressed that some patients may wish to know but not wish to talk about their condition, and that people of different social class and background may have different expectations and attitudes about the value of openness. It was admitted that in general it makes the minister's task much easier if the patient knows, but that he has no right to impose the truth on someone who does not ask or wish to know. ('Some people cannot stand too much reality. We have no right to break down their defences.') It was recognised that in general the minister must keep faith with the rest of the team if the agreed policy is not to tell, but that he should not be totally bound in conscience not to tell, if the patient asks and wishes to discuss it with him.

(vii) Different styles of spiritual ministry to the dying were discussed—Jewish, Catholic and Protestant—and much common ground discovered.

The Jewish traditions in the care of the dying were generally approved, namely: that the dying should not be left alone; that those staying with the dying should study the Bible and pray; that the dying should be encouraged to face the solemn moment with faith and courage, to set their worldly affairs in order, to offer forgiveness to those who had caused them hurt, to bless their children, and to make confession of their sins.

The administration of the sacraments (of Penance, Holy Communion and the Sacrament of the Sick) in the home and hospital was recognised as a means of bringing spiritual comfort to the dying, as a means of pointing them towards God and possibly helping them to accept the approach of death. These institutional forms were seen to have particular value in the hospital context where the privacy for intimate conversation might be lacking.

Although it was felt that the priest tends to be seen less as a harbinger of death, now that the Sacrament of the Sick is administered more frequently, it was recognised that the unexpected arrival of the priest could cause alarm.

The ministry of listening, of prayer and spiritual counsel were seen to have common importance for all believers. It was emphasised that the prime responsibility of the minister is to listen and to stay with the dying, to simply be with them. In addition the following points were stressed:

(a) that it should be recognised that people often have a need to express their anxieties about death and dying, that they should be given opportunity to talk, encouraged to express their real feelings, encouraged to explore what the experience means to them, encouraged to find their own sources of hope;

(b) that ministers should be prepared for the fact that people may, in addition to anxiety, express a great deal of Anger, Guilt, Remorse and Grief, that ministers should help people feel that it is safe to cry, to unload their pent-up feelings;

(c) that ministers should avoid being caught up in family conspiracies to bring spiritual comfort to those who don't want it and should make opportunity to be alone with the patient;

(d) that ministers should avoid giving empty reassurances, but should reassure patients in the hopes which they express themselves, that they can only point them towards God and encourage them to look forward to the coming change as a change for the better, reassure them that their families will be looked after;

(e) that even those who appear unconscious should not be left alone, should be spoken to, touched and reeassured;

(f) that unbelievers too may have a need of some outside person to speak to.

(f) *Areas of conflict with other professions*

(i) Lack of understanding of the role and responsibilities of funeral directors which gives rise to conflicts about times and arrangements for funerals, sometimes causing delay and distress to the family.

(ii) Post-mortems causing delays and uncertainty, additional distress to the family.

(iii) Over-sedation of the bereaved—when doctors yield to pressure from relatives—and the process of grieving cannot get started, when family are prevented from participating meaningfully in the funeral.

(iv) Disagreements with doctors and nurses as to whether people should be told—when there is a conspiracy of silence.

(v) Lack of co-operation in the sharing of essential information—when doctors and hospital staff keep the minister at arm's length.

(vi) Ignorance of the minister's role and possible function in the hospital or community team—when medical staff are indifferent to people's spiritual needs. (It was recognised that the minister has a duty to interpret that role to the doctor and others involved.)

(g) *Recommendations for improved training of clergy*

(i) It was emphasised that the changing pattern of mortality tends to make death more hidden, as it affects mainly the elderly and isolated. The education of attitudes to death has to begin with the recognition of the facts of death and bereavement. Ministers have a responsibility to know the facts and make them known, to make the community more aware of the needs of the dying and the bereaved.

(ii) Ordinary church teaching should not reflect the conspiracy of silence about death. Preparation for dying should begin when we are younger. The themes of Death and Resurrection, as also the reality of Suffering and Loss, should form part of the constant teaching of the Church as they are a constant part of life.

(iii) Customs such as kisting should possibly be encouraged, and churches might more commonly be made available for families to view the dead. The laity should be encouraged (as in the Jewish community) to become more involved in preparation for burial and the burial rites themselves, and in organising support for the bereaved, so that people in general may have a more realistic awareness of death and bereavement in society.

(iv) Trainee ministers should have the opportunity to meet and discuss with funeral directors the preparation of bodies for burial and the business and difficulties of funeral arrangements, before they have to assume responsibilities for funerals themselves.

(v) More emphasis should be placed on experientially based learning rather than academic training of ministers—particularly in contact with other professions (doctors, nurses, social workers and community workers) in the care of the suffering, needy, dying and bereaved. Hospitals or GP placements, visits to mortuaries, experience of counselling the bereaved (e.g. in CRUSE) should be encouraged.

(vi) In general ministers could benefit from pastoral experience under supervision—either under the supervision of expert pastoral trainers, or by attachment to another minister for a period. Proper de-briefing and opportunity for discussion is essential—particularly after harrowing experiences with the dying or distraught relatives.

(vii) There is a need for more on-going, in-service training of ministers, for example through extension of the present chaplaincy service. Ministers need to be better prepared and better informed to deal with the normal and pathological aspects of death and bereavement.

(viii) Ministers need to be encouraged to cultivate a deep and searching devotional life and a realistic openness to the reality of Death and Loss as well as the hope of the Resurrection.

Postscript. In spite of the acknowledgment that the work of Hinton (1967), Kübler-Ross (1970), Murray Parkes (1972), Cartwright, Hockey and Anderson (1973) and Lily Pincus (1974) and others are becoming more widely known by doctors, nurses, social workers and ministers, there was general agreement that far too little attention is given in training for these professions to the question of proper terminal care and the problems of the bereaved. It is certainly becoming more common for courses to be given on these subjects and for provision to be made for discussion of these issues in the training of health-care professionals, but the Working Group was convinced that this important field is still widely neglected in many areas and more detailed theoretical and practical training is necessary if the general standards of the care of the dying and the bereaved is to be improved. In addition it was felt that there is room for the education of public attitudes to death and dying—both at school and through the media—so that the community at large can be helped to recognise its responsibilities to the dying and the bereaved.

Social Work Viewpoint

The Social Workers' sub-group discussed the following issues: (a) what circumstances justify a social worker becoming involved in the care of the dying and the bereaved; (b) the nature of the social worker's role and responsibilities in the care of the dying and bereaved; (c) the main social work values which are relevant here; (d) areas of recurrent conflict with other professions.

Report and recommendations

The following main issues were discussed: (a) social work intervention, (i) in the community, (ii) in the hospital; (b) responsibilities to the dying and the bereaved; (c) values relevant to the care of the dying and the bereaved; (d) areas of recurrent conflict with other professions; (e) role of the social worker in the hospital setting; (f) education and training.

(a) SOCIAL WORK INTERVENTION

In the community. Social workers tend to become involved with the dying or the bereaved only where they have had previous contact with the individual/individuals concerned. When social workers have been involved in helping an individual or family with specific practical or social problems they tend to become further involved with other and more general problems of the individual or family concerned, including support for the dying or the bereaved. 'It's you being there and your past links that explain how you become involved. They give you the right. The client legitimates your involvement.'

Social workers tend to become involved with the dying when the circumstances of the death are abnormal or cause abnormal stress (e.g. the death of a child, or a difficult situation involving an elderly patient). Similarly sw's tend to become involved with the bereaved when there is an abnormal grief reaction which affects the ability of the individual to cope and causes concern to others or fear that someone may be put at risk. (The appropriateness of the person closest to be the one that gives the help was recognised, and it was admitted that the sw is rarely in that position. However, the sw gets drawn in when those nearest and dearest can't cope, when the situation becomes abnormal.)

In the hospital. It was recognised that in the hospital or institutional setting the sw may acquire responsibility in the care of the dying or their relatives because that responsibility is given them by the Medical Care Team. As the 'outside arm' of the hospital team and as the non-sepcific generalist the sw tends to be allocated the supportive role. 'That Medical Social Workers become involved in giving support to the dying and the bereaved is due to the fact that they form part of the caring service offered to people in touch with a modern hospital.' 'Although the Medical and Nursing staff take on part of the role what is specific about Social Work is its extension into the family. The cut-off point for the other professions is related to the completion of their specific tasks and comes sooner.'

(b) RESPONSIBILITIES

There was general agreement that it is not possible to separate the sw's responsibilities to the dying from responsibility to the bereaved. 'It's all grief-work. Helping the dying and the bereaved is helping them come to terms with loss. The dying are thinking about separating themselves from the living. Preparing someone for a 'good death' is a matter of preparing them for the final loss. Helping people face the possibility of death at an unknown time in the future is a matter of encouraging them to achieve a better quality of life rather than mere extension of life. There is a need for them to take a hold on the fact of death before they can get on with living. Fear, unresolved grief, panic, can overcome the will to live.' It was emphasised that in geriatric wards and old folks' homes people want to know about death, want to discuss it. They are all involved in the death of one member, all are bereaved. They want to know: What's it like? When's it my turn? They want information, otherwise they are left with their illusions and phantasies and the guilt that goes around. They have a need to share it, discuss it when someone dies.' 'I see people bereaved when the patient goes into hospital. The process of bereavement for patient and relatives begins then. My work begins then.' In general it was felt that the sw has the following responsibilities:

(i) To encourage as much openness about death as is compatible with the specific needs of the individual.

(ii) To encourage people to mourn and to mourn in the way they feel most appropriate.

(iii) To give people the opportunity to get out their pent-up feelings of grief, remorse, anger, fear and to help them accept that they have such feelings.

(iv) 'We should be involved in helping people, training people, to be in control of their own death—the alternative is that people give way to panic or despair.'

(v) To be prepared to share emotion with the client. 'When this mother's child died all I could do was cuddle her and let her cry and cry. That probably wasn't very professional behaviour, but it helped a lot.'

(vi) To be aware of the protracted nature of grief reactions in many cases, and to be available to come in 'when years later grief comes out'. 'It's a matter of sharing pain, of allowing pain to come out, often long after the event.' (It was agreed that the literature on Bereavement and Death—e.g. Hinton, Murray Parkes, Lily Pincus, is valuable, but that its relevance tends to be perceived only when the sw has been through the experience with a client.)

(c) VALUES

The specific values in Social Work, with application to the care of the dying and the bereaved, which were mentioned were:

(i) An emphasis on the value of truthfulness and openness, and a willingness to accept things as they are. 'The sw cannot operate without the pre-supposition of openness and equal access to information. Equally the sw may use this "demand for honesty" as a tool to manipulate doctors and the Medical Team.' ('Medical staff tend to "wrap things up". One feels disadvantaged as a sw. Are there different work values, or are we just "out of phase" with medical and nursing staff at certain times?')

(ii) An emphasis on the right of people to determine their own lives, their own mode of dying (sw's feel that people must, so far as possible, have the power to help themselves. The sw's philosophy is to facilitate self-determination, to encourage people to accept responsibility for their own lives. This is why (to doctors and nurses) they may often appear to be doing nothing.')

(iii) An emphasis on the right of disadvantaged and helpless people to proper advocacy, to proper representation of their interests and needs. ('The people we deal with are lacking in power, are usually not independent. Therefore they need help because they are not capable of helping themselves. Openness safeguards their interests too as it prevents sw's arrogating too much power to themselves.' 'sw's have a listening role—this contrasts with the tendency of doctors to prescribe answers.')

(iv) The sw tends to be concerned with the continuum of care in the community (sw's often have difficulties in knowing what limits to set to involvement, because they are concerned with people's social needs, therefore specific contracts need to be negotiated with clients.' 'Doctors are not trained to accept total social responsibility for patients and tend to see their role as specific to an individual and their medical problem.')

(d) CONFLICT WITH OTHER PROFESSIONS

With doctors: Conflicts over truth-tellıng in relation to patients with fatal conditions; conflicts over patient's rights—the right to die and the right to mourn. ('Doctors are often opposed to patients going home—say they will die quicker. The s w has to plead the right of the patient to go home to die if they want to.'); conflicts over the limits of confidentiality—the right of the patient to know—the right of other concerned individuals and professions ('Whose is the confidentiality? Whose truth is it?')

With nurses: 'sw's wish fervently that nurses would take more responsibility to tell. They are often the most appropriate person to do so, but refuse to do so because doctor, patient and other nurses don't expect it of them.'

(e) ROLE IN THE HOSPITAL SETTING

The social workers in hospital should function as an external arm of the institution, bringing into the treatment centre knowledge of the patient's normal response to stress, his significant relationships, his functioning in society—this with a view to personalising the service and helping the hospital staff understand the roots of his behaviour in the ward, in particular his emotional response to an alien setting. She must reflect the patient's real environment, including its strengths, as a means of counteracting dependency. She has a role in communicating the changing needs of relatives to medical staff, e.g. the wife who initially does not wish to discuss her husband's terminal prognosis but then reviews her decision. The social worker has knowledge of the services and resources available in the community to individuals and families coping with illness or adapting and adjusting to the changes in daily life necessitated by handicap or chronic illness.

With geriatric patients, she can help families mourn at admission to long-stay care; to express feelings about deterioration/change of personality in a loved one and about the condition and behaviour of other patients; and to cope with procedures. She assumes the role of catalyst for release of tensions in the family group so that the relatives can 'let go' without rejecting the patient.

(f) EDUCATION AND TRAINING

At present there is little evidence of teaching focusing specifically on the needs of the dying in basic social work training courses. However, there is considerable emphasis on the concepts of Attachment and Loss and their significance for human growth and behaviour, which ought to be readily transferable into work with the dying and the bereaved. (*Note*: CCETSW have just instituted a postqualifying course at Southampton University on Social Work with the elderly.)

Social work education and training should include Grief and Mourning Theory complemented by application in practice, since the learning will be integrated only when the experience has been confronted and then the theory reviewed. Anticipatory work would seem to be essential, with students thinking themselves into the patient's situation. Students need to be helped to examine their own attitudes and experiences, to confront their fears, anxieties and fantasies and to be in touch with their own feelings so that these do not block out the patient's reality. This work should be done so far as possible with other professionals in training.

Appendix 2

The critical perspective of Cruse, Funeral Directors and the Bereaved

THIS APPENDIX contains reports from three local bodies which co-operated with the EMG Research Project on Professional Attitudes and Values in the Care of the Dying and the Bereaved.

In the case of the report and recommendations of the Edinburgh, Lothian and Border Funeral Directors' Association this was drawn up after several meetings of the members at which they were asked to comment critically on the difficulties they experienced in present provisions and professional services to the dying and the bereaved.

The CRUSE recommendations were produced through a number of discussions with the EMG Project Research Staff and more particularly in discussions among the case-workers, rota helpers, staff and widows associated with CRUSE (Edinburgh Branch).

The observations and recommendations of the Widows, Widowers and Bereaved Parents Group (together with the comments from CRUSE) to represent a 'consumers' point of view on the weaknesses and deficiencies in present provisions for the care of the dying and the bereaved.

Edinburgh, Lothians and Border Funeral Directors' Association
Death and bereavement: recommendations for improvement of services
1. People need to be better informed about and prepared for death, specifically in relation to the following: ignorance of the complications which arise when people do not make provision for their death, e.g. when someone dies intestate; ignorance of medico-legal requirements when death occurs, ignorance regarding certification and registration of a death; ignorance regarding the need for medical investigation if the cause of death is uncertain; ignorance of the need for police investigation in the case of sudden, accidental or violent death; ignorance of what to do in relation to Insurance, Social Security, Death Grants, etc.
2. *Certification and Registration of Deaths*
(i) The recommendation of the Broderick Report regarding the simplification of procedures for certification and registration of deaths should be fully implemented. Doctors and hospital staff should be made conversant with the recommendations and present requirements. (E.g. Doctors should be made aware that Form C may be filled in by any doctor of 5 years standing. It is not necessary for a consultant to sign. Doctors and nurses should know that the relatives may register a death either in the place where death occurred or in the deceased's own place of residence.

Ignorance of these provisions or failure to inform relatives correctly can cause delays, unnecessary expense and travel, and general distress to people who are often elderly and poor as well as bereaved.)

O   189

(ii) It should be impressed on doctors and pathologists that possession of the right certificates is very important to the relatives and essential before arrangements for burial or cremation can be undertaken. Delays and confusion in relation to the procedure of certification of a death are a frequent cause of distress and anxiety to the bereaved and a source of much frustration to the funeral directors who cannot begin to make arrangements, contact relatives or announce a death until the formalities are completed.

(iii) Relatives are often inadequately briefed by hospital staff as to what they must do once they have the death certificate. In particular many are unaware that the registrar will give them a Form 14 in lieu of the death certificate so that they can proceed with other arrangements. Relatives ought to be instructed to have available the deceased's birth certificate for registration purposes.

(iv) Unnecessary delays are caused by virtue of the fact that fiscal's offices, mortuaries, crematoria and some doctors observe a 5-day week. If death occurs on a Friday afternoon or over a week-end there can be considerable and distressing delays caused simply because the necessary documents are not available to enable relatives and funeral director to proceed with arrangements. Relatives often have to be contacted twice—once to be informed of the death and a second time to confirm the date of the funeral—causing extra expense, and distress.

(v) The fact that certificates are filled out illegibly and signatures are illegible can also cause unnecessary delays (and prevent prompt payment of doctors too).

(vi) Doctors ought to be briefed to explain the cause of death to the relatives in simple and accurate terms, to avoid confusion and anxiety.

3. *Post-mortem*

(i) Are all PM's strictly necessary?—particularly in the case of infants, still-births and elderly people?

Relatives are often distressed at being approached to give permission for a PM. Relatives are often inadequately informed about the reasons for a PM being necessary. When there are medico-legal reasons for a PM particular tact should be shown in handling relatives.

(ii) Pathologists often make unnecessary incisions and cosmetic restoration can be badly done. This causes difficulty and embarrassment to the funeral director in preparing the corpse for viewing and causes unnecessary distress to relatives who come to pay their last respects to a beloved relative and wish to see them for the last time.

(iii) Indecisions about PM's can lead to unnecessary moving about of the remains from hospital to funeral parlour to mortuary, to funeral parlour, etc.—causing considerable delay and expense.

(iv) Medical indifference about still-births results in insensitivity to the need for proper certification/delivery notes to be completed expeditiously.

4. *Death grants and death on social security*

(i) Death grants, fixed at £20 in 1948, later increased by £10, are hopelessly inadequate. Should they be made payable to the person ordering the funeral? (The money is often spent on paying electricity or gas bills and not death expenses.)

(ii) The regionalisation of social services has complicated the procedure for claiming assistance where someone dies who has been living on social security. These procedures could be streamlined.

5. *General*

(i) Solicitors could take a more positive part in advising people to make adequate provision for their death.

(ii) Ministers are often difficult to contact and are often altogether inaccessible on Mondays.

(iii) Doctors, nurses and other hospital staff often show inadequate consideration to the bereaved and other family members in dealing with the practical details in the immediate aftermath of a death.

(iv) The errors and omissions of the Press in the publication of death notices can be a cause of embarrassment and distress to the family.

(v) Younger medical staff show scant respect for funeral directors and their staff and can be less than helpful with arrangements for the removal of remains.

The trend in Scotland tends to be away from people being directly involved in the laying out of their dead, or having the body on view in the house. The funeral director is expected to assume an ever-increasing responsibility in supporting and advising the bereaved famliy, and to act as a shock-absorber and intermediary between the bereaved and other professions and authorities.

Note: The following are some of the certificates which may be required at the time of a death:

Form A: Application for permission to cremate;

Form B: Medical Certificate of patient's doctor or G P;

Form C: Confirmatory Certificate by second doctor;

Form D: Pathologist's certificate in the case of a post-mortem examination;

Form E: Coroner's/Fiscal's certificate—in the case of a sudden death;

Form 14: Certificate given by the Registrar of Births, Deaths, etc. in lieu of the Death Certificate, which is retained by the Registrar.

Extracts of the Death Certificate showing primary and secondary cause of death can be obtained on payment from Registrar. (These extracts required for legal, insurance and banking purposes—being proof of death.)

Widows, Widowers and Bereaved Parents Group

1. *The hospital doctor*. There is a need for doctors to tell the truth and not side-step issues, especially in dealing with close relatives. There is need for continuity, both of information received, but more important, of the person seen. More co-ordination and discipline is necessary in the hospital scene if this continuity is to be possible and real understanding and sympathy built up between doctor, patient and relatives. There is a need to define when there is no point in going on with investigations and treatment, so that relatives are not left under any illusions about the uselessness of continuing treatment when there is no hope.

The comfort of receiving a letter from the hospital staff was emphasised, and it was also acknowledged that doctors and staff appreciate some feedback on how relatives are getting on.

Communication between hospital consultants and G Ps leaves a lot to be desired. There are unnecessary delays. The G P is often in possession of inadequate information to deal with the enquiries of patients and relatives.

Hospitals could do more to educate G Ps in the management of the dying—particularly in relation to appropriate dosages of pain-killing and other drugs, and in advising on the availability of professional help and technical aids. (It is often left to the relatives to complain and this complicates relations with G Ps.)

2. *General practitioners*. There is a need for closer co-operation between G P, hospital and relatives over the moving of elderly sick patients into hospital, or from one hoapital to another. Relatives are not always informed in advance when patients are to be moved. It tends to be at the convenience of the ambulance men or hospital, and often at the expense of the patient and his needs. The consequence is that relatives are unable to assist adequately in preparing elderly patients for moves and changes—whieh causes greater confusion,

disorientation and distress than is necessary (and in some cases results in the premature death of the patient).

Both elderly patients and very young children are liable to be distressed by the change from supervision by a familiar G P to a strange hospital doctor or doctors; and by loss of contact with 'their doctor'. Sudden switches in ward staff dealing with elderly patients also caused distress and added confusion. Children too tended to become very attached to 'their staff' and were upset by changes. In dealing with the terminally ill, change and dislocation ought to be avoided so far as possible.

The hospital visit from the G P was greatly appreciated by the patient and the relatives. It was regretted that more G Ps do not visit their patients in hospital, especially when they are dying.

It was felt by all to be important that GPs should be more frank in communicating prognoses, especially when the outcome was likely to be fatal. Reservations were expressed in some exceptional cases. It was maintained that GPs tend to err on the side of caution and 'are inclined to treat people like children'. Responsible and adult people need time to sort out their affairs, relationships and personal attitudes, and perhaps to share their bereavement with their spouse or family. Not being told deprives them of their opportunity.

8. *Nurses.* It was felt that nurses tend to edge relatives out, want to get them out of the way. This leaves relatives feeling useless and unwanted, whereas there are many things they can do to help. Nurses should be trained to get the relatives to help, to encourage them to assist as much as possible with minor nursing tasks. Relatives (especially in the home) may need to be taught simple but necessary skills and what aids to use so that they can help effectively.

While it was recognised that some relatives cannot cope and are distressed by seeing, e.g. injections being given, in general it was felt that with terminal patients it is very important for the patient and the relatives that the latter should be given the opportunity to help.

While it was recognised that district nurses are more likely than hospital nurses to allow the relatives to share simple nursing tasks, it was also felt that if two nurses attend together they tend to take over and push the family out. There is a tendency for the DN to feel that she must do something or her visit is wasted, whereas reassurance and encouragement to the family that they are managing well may be all that is needed.

It was felt that hospital nurses are often not sufficiently well informed about the specific needs of the dying patient and his family and tend therefore to react inappropriately. Better briefing of nurses would remove uncertainty and perhaps help to reduce anxiety at ward level—as nurses would be better equipped to deal with enquiries from other patients. On the whole it was felt that everyone in the ward should know, if possible.

It was felt that it should not be the responsibility of the nurse to tell the dying patient, but that relatives should be encouraged to do so if the patient wanted to know their condition. It was recognised that if people are to be told the truth there is a need for a whole terminal care set-up and a supporting community.

There is a need for some specific individual or class of individual in a hospital to be properly trained and charged with the responsibility for giving bereaved relatives immediate help and practical assistance. (Question: Whether the No. 7, senior ward sister, would not be the appropriate person.) People need practical advice on death procedure and nurses should be able to give this.

There is need for much greater care in the delivery of death messages. The phone call simply saying that So-and-so had died is quite the wrong thing. Very much better would be a message to the police or to some other person in the community who could quietly tell the relative face to face and ensure that they are not left alone afterwards.

In relation to bereaved relatives it was maintained that all too often the nurses give the patient's relatives a cup of tea and then send them on their way without enquiring whether they have someone to drive them home or have anyone to go to. It was emphasised that people should be discouraged from driving themselves home, that if possible arrangements should be made so that bereaved persons are not left on their own.

4. *Social workers and other hospital staff.* While it was felt that social workers have perhaps little part to play at the moment of death, it was felt that they could be of great assistance in helping relatives when they are told bad news—either when coping with the shock of a fatal diagnosis, or in coping with immediate grief-reactions.

It was felt that sws have a lot of experience of dealing with people facing various kinds of loss and that they could be very helpful in the follow-up of bereaved people—particularly where the bereavement is protracted or where the death causes serious complications to the life of relatives.

Ambulancemen it was agreed can play a key role in the initial crisis situation, and can be very helpful and supportive, or the converse. Hospital technicians and even hospital porters can give great assistance to the dying and their relatives.

As regards giving 'human' help and support, almost any member of the hospital staff who is prepared to be understanding can be of assistance at a time of death and bereavement. Hospital staff should be alerted to this possibility.

Geographical considerations: It was noted that there can be much greater problems involved when people die at a distance from home, or abroad, and that officials show lack of appreciation of the need of bereaved relatives for practical assistance and advice.

5. *Funeral directors.* Funeral directors gave invaluable advice and practical assistance—especially if they did not appear too busy, rushed and 'efficient'.

There were sometimes special difficulties with sudden death in the home, where death tended to be more untidy, where a second medical opinion might have to be sought, and FDs were unwilling or unable to get involved.

Funeral directors seemed to be at their best in dealing with other professions in the hospital context and were particularly good at facilitating things for the family when it came to dealing with hospitals and hospital red tape. They appeared to be less at ease in dealing with the more intimate and delicate situation of death in the home.

People should be encouraged to discuss arrangements for their burial or cremation in a matter-of-fact and business-like way long before the event, and even to make provision for it by insurance or in their wills. Lawyers and funeral directors could help to de-mystify death by encouraging people to make proper advance arrangements and make their intentions known so that shocked and bereaved relatives would not be left to make painful decisions in uncertain circumstances.

The innovation of recent 'Peace-of-mind' insurance policies was thought to be a good thing and the question was asked whether funeral directors should not more actively offer an advisory service to the living.

6. *Teachers and schools.* The role of teachers and schools can be crucial in helping or hindering the child who has lost a parent. Teachers need to be alerted to the following situations where they need great tact and sensitivity: (a) where they have to break the news to the child or children; (b) where the child may have a strong emotional attachment to his teacher and particularly needs that teacher to acknowledge his concern and awareness of the child's

grief; (c) where the bereaved child needs to be helped to be reintegrated into the class after an absence following a death, and needs the teacher's help to get the class to recognise his problem and his loss; (d) where the child develops behaviour problems due to acute anxiety and insecurity and may need special attention or help; (e) where the class may need opportunity to talk out its shock or grief reactions—where there has been a sudden, accidental or violent death.

7. *The social stigma of mental illness—dementia and death.* The need for hospital and medical staff to be more sensitive to the problems of relatives whose loved ones die or are dying in mental hospitals. The need for the education of public attitudes towards psycho-geriatric and mentally ill patients—especially those dying demented.

There needs to be recognition of the peculiar distress, humiliation and often prolonged bereavement of those cut off from their dying relatives by their madness. The case of the 'widow' whose husband is still alive, but demented.

The peculiar problems of children whose memories of a parent are unhappy and hate-filled—because of their madness and the violence which may have been associated with it, causing irrational fear and inability to understand.

8. *Parents, children and 'death education'.* Strongly divergent views were expressed about the exposure of children to death, corpses, funerals and overt manifestations of bereavement. There were also sharp differences over the values of 'death education'—e.g.: encouraging children to talk about a death that affects them, giving information about social customs, ritual and death procedure, or encouraging attendance at funerals, or visits to cemeteries and crematoria. The value of sharing a bereavement with one's children was acknowledged, and the comforting role children could play, recognised.

It was generally admitted that the greatest help at the time of bereavement tended to come from the family, and others who were also affected, that there was great help in knowing the ropes, knowing what had to be done, how, when and where. There is a need for people to be better informed about what to do when death occurs, and what help they can get.

It was felt that while children may appear to have a more basic, natural and realistic view of death and may appear better able to accept death at the time, the real impact of a bereavement on a child may only show up years later. Adults may appear to grieve more deeply, but may also get over bereavement more quickly and more completely. The loss of a parent may only show itself later in the child in odd adolescent behaviour. A mother cannot make up for the loss of the influences of a father in the life of a child—and there can be problems with step-dads.

9. *Priests and ministers.* It was generally acknowledged that, even for non-believers, the ministry of a concerned clergyman could be of great value, not in an officious clerical role, but (because of their familiarity with death) for the practical advice and assistance they could give, by being willing to be there and to listen, and in simply representing faith and hope—not necessarily talking about it.

It was recognised that there is much in common in the kind of ministry offered to the dying and the bereaved by the clergy of the different churches. However, it was felt that there are some interesting differences between the approach of Protestant ministers and Episcopalian and Catholic priests. It was felt that the Protestant minister tends to approach the patient or family more as an individual and the effectiveness of his ministry seems to be more dependent on the personality of the individual man and his personal availability, though he is also there to represent the Church and the resources of the Church. The Catholic priest, whose ministry need be no less personal, operates within a more institutionalised framework where provision is made for the administration of the sacraments, where people expect the service of a priest and where priests are perhaps more readily available. It was suggested that the sacramental ministry of Episcopal and Catholic clergy perhaps fits in more naturally with hospital medicine but the supportive and counselling role of other clergy is just as important if not more so, but more difficult to exercise in a hospital ward. Neither approach helps everyone, but each has its advantages and disadvantages. People do seem to need to rationalise, make sense of, the experience of death or bereavement. Having beliefs seems to help—even if only in providing a framework of rules within which to continue living and attempting to cope. For many the experience of bereavement was associated with loss of faith, for some it was recovered and strengthened.

CRUSE: Notes and Recommendations
1. *Before the death of the patient*
(a) *Communication between medical staff and patient and his family.* There is need for as much frankness and honesty as possible—confusion results otherwise. Difficulties are more likely to arise when the doctor and relatives don't know each other, and with change of personnel. Even if the doctor judges that the patient should not be told that he is dying *it is imperative that the family should be told.* Hospital staffs sometimes seem too liable to treat relatives as less than intelligent adults, and consequently the relatives may respond as such.

People can be left with feelings of guilt for not being sympathetic enough because they didn't know the patient was dying. Telling the patient depends on individual cases. Whatever one thinks in theory, the situation can be different in practice.

If a doctor says that a patient has not got cancer when he has, this can produce a subsequent lack of trust of the medical profession as a whole.

The great increase in early diagnosis raises more queries from patients and relatives, and doctors should learn how to cope with this situation. They should have opportunities to talk things through with patients and families. Perhaps the Group could find ways to help the doctors to organise this, and make specific recommendations to training bodies in this regard.

Student nurses should not be the ones to have to tell of the diagnosis, nor of the fact of death. There should be some specific appointment for the job—some experienced person who can talk to people on a one-to-one basis. We stress the importance of this person being available particularly at night, and that accommodation appropriate for this type of interview should be provided.

(b) *Care-sharing on the ward.* The current trend in society seems to be to isolate the dying patient, and relatives often experience feelings of lack of sufficient contact and communication with the hospital authorities. Taking the example of the modern children's ward, where mothers often help in the general care of the children, we suggest a move towards a similar situation in hospitals, whereby the dying person's relative would give similar assistance, e.g. feeding, being with, hand-holding, etc. Such a development could go some way towards breaking down the mystique about death, be a considerable comfort to the dying person and reduce the feeling of helplessness felt by so many relatives. There are obvious difficulties to be overcome in such a development, and all relatives would not necessarily be able or willing to participate in this way, but perhaps it is something which might be considered. This is already being done in some countries, e.g. Italy and Africa.

(c) *Psychiatric hospitals.* Particular problems arise when the dying person is mentally ill. Sometimes relatives are afraid of making a fuss based on anything the patient may have said, (a) because staff might 'take it out on him' and (b) because credence may not be placed on anything that he may have said. The attitude of nurses to mentally ill patients seems to be different to that to the physically ill. They can appear incapable of giving support to bereaved relatives because they assume that death is a release both to the patient and to the relative. While this may be true, the wife still suffers bereaved reactions. There are difficulties also in the attitude of the general public, and difficulties in talking things over with the children. Mrs S. was allowed to sit with her husband when he was in a coma, but nothing was said to her after his death. It was just assumed to be a release on both sides. She never saw any social worker.

Note: This experience was not recent; things may have improved since then. Perhaps psychiatrists and nursing staff in mental hospitals are not as familiar with death as are those in general hospitals, and need more help in understanding relatives' reactions.

We have had requests from wives whose husbands are in long-stay and mental hospitals who regard themselves as virtual widows, and share the same difficulties as those who are in fact bereaved.

(d) *Hospital chaplains.* The experience of the group has been that visits by some hospital chaplains to dying patients have not always been helpful. It would be beneficial if people could work towards more relevant consultation between hospital chaplains, hospital staff and the relatives before visits are made.

2. *Post bereavement*

(a) *Death messages.* Although it was felt important not to delay news of a death, it is very undesirable that the hospital should ring up and give the message to someone alone in the house; but impossible to ask if they are alone and not say anything if so. We endorse this as an area to be given greater consideration. This, presumably, would come within the remit of the 'specific appointment' (see 1(a)).

Perhaps the hospital could make a note of the next-but-one of kin, as well as the next of kin—or some nearby relation—or of all the family. Or more use might be made of the police to give the information.

It should not be left to a junior nurse to give the message. Young people can't be expected to know how to cope unless given some instruction and help.

At a recent day study, of a group of about 40 doctors, nurses, clergy, social workers, etc. (age group 30s-50s) only one, a recently qualified social worker, had had anything about bereavement in his/her training.

(b) *Deaths of children and grandchildren.* We question the 'shielding' of children and keeping them away from the realities of death and mourning. The whole family should share in the grief thus supporting each other by everyone's affection. Guilt feelings in children are very frequent when this does not happen, but instance was given of a young boy after viewing the body of his friend who died after an asthma attack saying 'Now I know it wasn't anything I had done that made him die.' When a young person dies someone should watch out for the reactions (often delayed) of the other siblings. Important that their teachers know of their bereavement.

(c) *Post mortems.* Requests for post mortems can be terribly distressing for the relatives, and medical staff should be given help in knowing the best way to communicate the reasons for these procedures. There seems to be a difference when the reasons are medical rather than legal, and the knowledge that the post mortem may benefit future generations—be 'an investment in the future'—may make the idea seem more acceptable. It has been found that the police are generally very good when the necessity is a legal one.

(d) *Drugs.* While we recognise the value of medication, sustained personal support can be as beneficial. Doctors are sometimes inclined to push medication; indiscriminate prescribing should be avoided. GPs should be on the look

196

out for *extreme, prolonged* or *delayed* reactions, warning signals that something may be wrong in the natural grieving process.

A family doctor will often visit a bereaved person within the first few days, and this visit can be much appreciated. We suggest that some consideration be given to making a habit of a follow-up visit, say in six weeks, by either the doctor or health visitor, and that all medical staff should be alerted to the possibility of problem reactions.

(c) *Dying at home.* Family doctors are usually involved pretty soon anyway. There is more scope for a personal relationship in these circumstances, and assessment by the doctor of the situation. The professional is on the relatives' territory, not vice versa, and this can make the relationship more natural from the relatives' point of view.

(f) *Hospital funerals.* There is a good case for the provision of facilities for a brief and simple hospital funeral in the case of still-births, and also in the case where the body is donated for medical research. (In the former case if there has to be a PM the delay can be distressing and the formalities of a full-scale funeral unnecessarily harrowing. In the latter case although the remains are buried eventually, there is no clear cut-off point for the bereaved unless there is some suitable ceremony.)

(Sgd.) M. Cowan (*Secretary*)
CRUSE (Edinburgh Branch)
April 1977

Acknowledgments

THIS STUDY of Professional Attitudes and Values in the Care of the Dying and the Bereaved was undertaken as part of the Edinburgh Medical Group Research Project in Medical Ethics and Education. The research project was set up by generous grants from the Nuffield Provincial Hospitals Trust and from the Leverhulme Trust Fund, with the twin objectives of exploring the possibility of multi-disciplinary research in medical ethics and its relevance and application to education and training in the health-care professions.

In setting up the Working Group the EMG Research Staff received helpful advice from a number of people. In particular the staff wish to thank the Chairman of their Steering Committee, Sir Michael Swann, and its members, Mr T. D. Hunter, Professor R. H. Girdwood, The Revd D. W. D. Shaw, Miss L. Hockey, Professor A. S. Duncan, Professor A. P. M. Forrest, Professor R. V. Short, Dr B. Potter, Dr G. Wright, Revd Dr K. M. Boyd, Dr L. Gruer, Miss E. Scott and Mrs A. Wolf. In this context the gratitude of the Edinburgh Medical Group as a whole must be expressed for the contribution of the late Professor James Blackie, without whose work and encouragement as Chairman of the Consultative Council and Joint Grant Holder, the EMG Project would not have come into existence.

The Research Staff are particularly grateful to the individual members of the Working Group for their enthusiastic participation in this two-year research project and for their generous sacrifice of time in preparing papers and cases for discussion and attending many meetings. However, it may be felt that formal thanks are not necessary, for, as many members have remarked, the participation in such an exercise, like the practice of virtue, is its own reward. It was by common consent an invaluable learning experience and while it might be difficult to communicate its precise significance, it was hoped that its benefits would be shown in increased understanding and sensitivity in professional practice and inter-professional relationships in the care of the dying and the bereaved.

Acknowledgments

Research Staff
Chairman: Dr D.O.Edge, Director, University of Edinburgh Science Studies Unit
Nuffield Research Fellow: Dr I.E.Thompson, former lecturer in Philosophy
Medical Adviser: Dr C.T.Currie, Lecturer in Geriatric Medicine
Nursing Adviser: Dr A.J.Tierney, Lecturer in Nursing Studies

Working Group Members
Miss S.Bett: District Nurse and Matron of Marie Curie Hospital, Springburn, Glasgow
Miss M.Buchanan: Principal Nursing Officer, Royal Hospital for Sick Children, Edinburgh
Mr J.T.Cameron, QC: Advocate and Legal Adviser
Dr J.J.C.Cormack: General Practitioner, Corstorphine, Edinburgh
Miss M. Coverdale: Social Worker, Development Officer for Age Concern, Scotland
Dr A.C.Douglas: Consultant Physician, Department of Respiratory Diseases
Dr D.Doyle: Medical Director, St Columba's Hospice, Edinburgh
Mrs I.Duncan: Social Worker, Department of Geriatric Medicine
Professor A.P.M.Forrest: Department of Clinical Surgery, Edinburgh
Mr S.Guild, WS: Solicitor and Legal Adviser to CRUSE
Miss L.Hockey: Director, University of Edinburgh Nursing Studies Research Unit
Dr C.P.Lowther: Consultant Physician, Department of Geriatric Medicine
Revd T.S.McGregor: Chaplain, Royal Infirmary, Edinburgh
Mrs M.MacKay: Area Officer, Musselburgh Social Work Team
Miss J.MacKenzie: Ward Sister, Radiotherapy Unit, Western General Hospital
Mrs J.Meikle: District Nurse, formerly with Group Practice attachment in Edinburgh
Dr B.Potter: recently qualified Junior Hospital Doctor
Dr E.B.Ritson: Consultant Psychiatrist, Royal Edinburgh Hospital

During the course of its deliberations the Working Group was assisted and advised by a number of representatives of local organisations and other professional and lay people. To all these we owe a debt of thanks:

First, we wish to thank Inspector Cameron and the Staff of the

Training Division of the Lothian and Borders Police, for the opportunity to consult them and their students about police training in the handling of sudden, accidental and violent death, and the giving of death messages to relatives.

Second, we are most grateful to Mrs Margaret Cowan and Mrs Una Armour of CRUSE (Edinburgh Branch), and to the caseworkers, rota-helpers and widows who gave us valuable insight into the problems of the bereaved and the kinds of assistance which they can be given.

Third, we are indebted to Mr William Purves, President of the Edinburgh, Lothians and Borders Funeral Directors Association, and to all its members who assisted us with practical reflections on present services to the dying and the bereaved.

Fourth, we wish to thank Mr Ian Walker, WS, of the Samaritans, for his help and advice on legal issues which arise in connection with a death in the family.

Fifth, we are particularly grateful to all the widows, widowers and bereaved parents who, in the specially convened group under the chairmanship of Professor A.P.M. Forrest, met several times to prepare recommendations on the improvement of services to the dying and the bereaved. (The substance of what was gathered from the police, CRUSE, the funeral directors and the group of bereaved, is summarised in Chapter 3 and their recommendations are published in the Appendix.)

Dr C.M.U. Maclean and Revd Dr K.M. Boyd, who as guests presented papers to the Working Group, must be thanked for the way they helped to direct our thinking, especially in its early stages. Their two seminal papers have been published in the *Journal of Medical Ethics* (Boyd, K.M. (1977) Attitudes to death—some historical notes, Vol. 3, no. 3, and Maclean, C.M.U. (1979) Learning about Death Vol. 5, no. 2).

Various sub-groups were convened to formulate recommendations for education and training of health-care professionals in the care of the dying and the bereaved. Our special thanks are due to the chairman, Revd Dr A.V. Campbell and ministers of various denominations who participated in the Clergy sub-group, to the Social Workers from the Lothian Region who helped in the Social Workers' sub-group, and to the Doctors and Nurses who assisted in the Medical and Nursing sub-groups. (Their recommendations are also published in the Appendix to this report.)

An unexpected development of the Research Project—yet fully in line with its educational aims—was the co-operation of the Research Staff and members of the Working Group with the BBC Man Alive Report team in the making of a film about death and bereavement entitled: 'Nothing to be afraid about'. This film illustrated the general 'conspiracy of silence' about death and dying in society, the inadequacy of the preparation of doctors and nurses to deal with the problems of death and bereavement, the more realistic approach of police and funeral directors, the predicament of the elderly and the problems of isolation and stigmatisation among widows and other bereaved. The film was intended and has been extensively used as a teaching aid. For the opportunity of this co-operation with the BBC we are grateful to its Chairman, Sir Michael Swann, for it was at his suggestion that the making of this film was undertaken. We are also grateful to the Producer, David Filkin, for his skilful and sympathetic handling of such sensitive material.

Last, but not least, the Research Staff wish to thank the EMG Project Office Secretaries, Mrs Margaret Cowell and Mrs Maureen Bannatyne who minuted proceedings and who, together with Mrs Nan Hamilton, helped to type the various drafts of this report. Their untiring patience, good humour and efficiency considerably lightened the burden of the production of this book.

We are thus indebted to many people for their help and advice in conducting the research and in the preparation of this report. Aware that its imperfections are ours, we can only hope that it may do some justice to their concern with the ethics and practice of terminal care and care of the bereaved, that it may have some value as a source book for training health-care professionals, and that it may help to shape public opinion, and thus encourage improvement in care of the dying and the bereaved.

Selected Bibliography

Abrams, R. D. (1966) The patient with cancer, his changing pattern of communication. *New Eng. J. Med.* 274, 317–22.

Agate, J. (1973) Care of the dying in Geriatric Departments. *Lancet* (Feb. 17), 365–6.

—— Let me go in peace. *Doc. in Med. Ethics 1* (SSME).

Agee, J. (1967) *A Death in the Family.* New York: Grosset and Dunlap.

Aitken-Swan, J. (1959) Nursing the late cancer patient at home. *Practitioner* 183, 64–9.

Aldrich, C. K. (1963) The dying patient's grief. *J. of Am. Med. Assoc. 184.*

Anderson, E. R. (1973) The role of the nurse. *RCN Study of Nursing Care Project Reports 2 (1).* London.

Annas, G. J. (1974) Rights of the terminally ill patients. *J. of Nursing Adm.* 4 (2), 40–44.

Anthony, S. (1973) *The Discovery of Death in Childhood and After.* London: Penguin Books.

Aries, P. (1976) *Western Attitudes toward Death. From the Middle Ages to the Present.* (Tr. P. M. Ranussi.) Johns Hopkins Press.

Aristotle (1972) *Nichomachean Ethics.* (Tr. with Intro. by Sir D. Ross.) London: World Classics 546.

Ayd, F. J., Jr. (1962) The hopeless case: medical and moral considerations. *J. of the Am. Med. Assoc. 181,* 1099–102.

Bady, M. (1973) *Nursing and Social Change.* London: Heinemann.

Baker, A. A. (1976) Slow euthanasia — or 'She will be better off in hospital'. *B.M.J. 4,* 571–2.

Balint, M. (1957) (1974) *The Doctor, his Patient and the Illness.* London: Pitman Medical.

Ball, M. (1976) *Death,* Oxford Univ. Press.

Bard, B. & J. Fletcher. (1968) The right to die. *Atlantic Mag.,* 59–64.

Barnlund, D. C. (1976) The mystification of meanings: doctor-patient encounters. *J. of Med. Educ. 51,* 716–25.

Barton, D. (1972) Death and dying: a psychiatrist's perspective. *Soundings* 55, 459–71.

Batten, L. W. (1970) Terminal illness at home. *Nursing Times* (27 Feb.) 28.

Battin, A., *et al.* (1975) Telephone intervention in the therapy of bereaved families. *J. of Thanatol. 3,* 43–7.

Baughman, W. H. (1973) Euthanasia: criminal tort, constitutional and legislative questions. *Notre Dame Lawyer 48,* 1202–60.

Becker, D. P. *et al.* (1970) An evaluation of the definition of cerebral death. *Neurology 20,* 459–62.

Becker, E. (1973) *The Denial of Death.* New York: Free Press.

203

Selected Bibliography

Beecher, H. K. Ethical problems created by the hopelessly unconscious patient. *Doc. in Med. Ethics 2* (SSME).

Behnke, J. A. & S. Bok, eds (1975) *The Dilemma of Euthanasia*. New York: Anchor Press/Doubleday.

Bellis, G. H. (1977) Death is not the end of caring. *Midwife, Health Visitor and Community Nurse 13*.

Benjamin, M. (1976) Death, where is thy 'cause'? *Hastings Center Report 6/3*, 15.

Bennett, A. E., ed. (1976) *Communication between Doctors and Patients*. Published for Nuffield Provincial Hospitals Trust by Oxford University Press.

Benoliel, J. Q. (1970) Talking to patients about death. *Nursing Forum 9 (3)*.

—— (1971) Assessments of loss and grief. *J. of Thanatol. 3*, 182–95.

Bernstein, S. (1960) Self-determination: king or citizen in the realm of values. *Social Work (U.S.A.) 5 (1)*.

Biestek, F. (1957) *The Casework Relationship*. Chicago.

Biorck, G. (1967) On the definitions of death. *World Med. J. 14*, 137–9.

Birtchnell, J. *et al.* (1973) *Effects of Early Parent Death*. New York: MSS Information Corporation.

Black, D. (1976) Working with widowed mothers. *Social Work Today 6 (22)*.

Blackham, H. J., ed. Ethical standards in counselling. Papers presented by a Working Party to the Standing Conference for the Advancement of Counselling. London: Bedford Square Press.

Blewett, J. J. (1970) To die at home. *Am. J. of Nursing 70*, 2602–4.

Bloch, S. Instruction on death and dying for the medical student. *Jnl of Medical Education July 1976*, Vol. 10, No. 4.

Bok. S. *et al.* (1973) The dilemmas of euthanasia. *BioScience 23*, 461–78.

—— (1976) Personal directions for care at the end of life. *New Eng. J. Med. 295*, 367–9.

Boros, L. (1965–9) *The Moment of Truth: Mysterium Mortis*. London: Burns & Oates.

Bourne, G. & P. Lindley (1976) Suicide. *Nursing Mirror: 15 July*.

Boyd, K. (1977) Attitudes to death: some historical notes. *J. of Med. Ethics 3 (3)*.

Branson, R., *et al.* (1976) The Quinlan decision: five commentaries. *Hastings Center Report 6/1*, 8–23.

Briar, S. & Miller (1971) *Problems and Issues in Social Casework*. Columbia Univ. Press.

Brierley, J. B., *et al.* (1971) Neocortical death after cardiac arrest. *Lancet Sept. 11*, 560–5.

Brill, H. W. (1970) Death with dignity: a recommendation for statutory change. *University of Florida Law Review 12*, 368–83.

Brim, O. G., Jr., *et al.* (1970) *The Dying Patient*. New York: Russell Sage Foundation.

British Assoc. of Social Workers. (1971) *Confidentiality in Social Work*.

—— (1975) *A Code of Ethics for Social Work*. Clifton House, Euston Rd, London NW1 2RS.

British Medical Association (1974) *Medical Ethics*. London: B.M.A.

Brauer, P. (1965) Should the patient be told the truth? In *Social Interaction and Patient Care* (eds J. K. Skipper & P. C. Ward), pp. 167–78. Philadelphia: Lippicott.

Brody, H. (1974) Teaching medical ethics: future challenges. *J. Am. Med. Assoc. 229*, 177–9.

—— (1975) Integrating ethics into the medical curriculum: one school's progress report. *Michigan Medicine (Feb.)*, 111–17.

—— (1976) The physician-patient contract: legal and ethical aspects. *J. of Legal Med., July/Aug.,* 25–30.

Brothers, J. (1971) The role of the minister in *Religious Institutions* Ch. 5. London: Longman.

Brown, N., *et al.* (1970) The preservation of life. *J. of the Am. Med. Assoc. 221,* 76–82.

Bullough, B. (1976) The law and the expanding nursing role. *Am. J. of Public Health 66,* 249–54.

Bunch, B., *et al.* (1976) Dealing with death: the unlearned role. *Am. J. of Nursing 76 (9),* 1486–8.

Bunzl, M. (1975) A note on nursing ethics in the U.S.A. *J. of Med. Ethics 1/4,* 184.

Campbell, A. V. (1972) *Moral Dilemmas in Medicine.* Churchill Livingstone.

Cantor, N. L. (1972) A patient's decision to decline life-saving medical treatment: bodily integrity versus the preservation of life. *Rutgers Law Review 26,* 228–64.

Canvin, R. W. & J. M. Nerrell (1975) Care of the dying in Exeter. *Nursing Times* (12 June), 942–3.

Carlson, C. E. (1970) Grief and mourning, in *Behavioural Concepts and Nursing Intervention.* Philadelphia: Lippincott.

Carmody, J. (1974) *Ethical Issues in Health Services: A Report and Annotated Bibliography.* Washington D.C.: U.S. Dept. of Health, Education and Welfare, 55 pp.

Cartwright, A. (1967) *Patients and their Doctors.* London: Routledge.
—— *et al.* (1973) *Life Before Death.* London: Routledge.

Case Conference (1975) The limits of informed consent. *J. of Med. Ethics 1/3 Sept.,* 146.

Case Conference (1976) The limits of confidentiality. *J. of Med. Ethics 2/1 March,* 28.

Case Conference (1977) Death my only love. *J. of Med. Ethics 3 (2). June,* 93.

Case Study (1975) A demand to die. *Hastings Center Report.*

Cassels, E. J. (1969) Death and the physician. *Commentary, June,* 73–9.

Central Council for Education & Training in Social Work (1976) *Values in Social Work:* social work curriculum. *Study Paper 13.* London: C.C.E.T.S.W.

Choron, J. (1972) *Suicide.* New York: Scribner.
—— (1973) *Death and Western Thought.* New York: Collier Books.

Church of England Board for Social Responsibility (1975) *On Dying Well.* London: Church Information Office.

Clare, A. (1976) *Psychiatry in Dissent.* London: Tavistock Institute.

Clarke, D. D. & D. M. Clarke (1977) Definitions and ethical decisions. *J. Med. Ethics 3 (4).*

Clauser, K. D. & A. Zucker (1974) *Abortion and Euthanasia: An Annotated Bibliography.* Philadelphia Soc. for Health and Human Values.

Coggan, D. (1977) On Dying and dying well: extracts from the Edwin Stevens Lecture. *J. of Med. Ethics 3 (2).*

Collected Conference Papers (1971) *Death and Dying.* Sponsored by Catholic Hospital Assoc. and Inst. for Theological Encounter with Science and Technology. St Louis.

Conference of Medical Royal Colleges (1976) Diagnosis of brain death. *Lancet 2,* 1069–70.

Contact No. 12 (1964) Grief and mourning. *October.*
—— No. 18 (1966) The waiting room for death. *October.*
—— No. 38 (1972) The problem of euthanasia. *Summer.*

Selected Bibliography

Cramond, W. A. (1973) The psychological care of patients with terminal illness. *Nursing Times, 15 March,* 339–43.

Crane, D. (1969) The social aspects of the prolongation of life. *Social Science Frontiers.* New York: The Russell Sage Foundation.

—— (1975) *The Sanctity of Social Life: Physician's Treatment of Critically Ill Patients.* New York: Russell Sage Foundation.

Cranston, M. (1974) *What are Human Rights?* London: Bodley Head.

Crichton, I. (1976) *The Art of Dying.* London: Peter Owen.

Cronin, A. J. (1939) *The Citadel.* London: Gollancz.

Cutler, D., ed. (1969) *Updating Life and Death.* Boston: Beacon Press.

Dent, C. E. Some doctors' attitudes to euthanasia. *Doc. in Med. Ethics 1* (SSME).

Death Education. *Death Education* (An International Quarterly). Washington: Hemisphere Publishing Corp.

D'Entrevres, A. P. (1951) *Natural Law.* London: Hutchinson.

Dewi Rees, W. (1972) The distress of dying. *Br. Med. J. (July 8).*

—— Bereavement and illness (1972) *J. of Thanatol. 2* (3–4), 785–820.

Donald, I. Naught for your comfort. *Doc. in Med. Ethics 1* (SSME).

Douglas, J. D. (1967) *The Social Meaning of Suicide.* New Jersey: Princeton University Press.

Downie, P. A. (1974) A personal commentary on the care of the dying in the North American continent. *Nursing Mirror 139 (15),* 68–70.

Downie, R. S. (1971) *Roles and Values.* London: Methuen.

Downing, A. B., ed. (1969) *Euthanasia and the Right to Die.* London: Peter Owen.

Dunea, G. (1976) Death with dignity. *B.M.J., 3 April.*

Dunstan, G. R. Euthanasia: clarifying the issues. *Doc. in Med. Ethics 1* (SSME).

Duncan, A.S., Dunstan, G. R. & Welbourn, R. B. eds (1974) *Dictionary of Medical Ethics.* London: Darton, Longman & Todd.

Durkheim, E. (1952) Suicide: *A Study in Sociology.* London: Routledge.

Dryden, K. G. (1975) The deceased husband and the rights of the widow. *Queens Nursing J., Dec.,* 249.

Eadie, H. A. (1972) The health of Scottish clergymen. *Contact 41.*

—— (1973) Stress and the clergyman. *Contact 42.*

—— (1974) They're human too. *Contact 43.*

—— (1975) The helping personality. *Contact 49.*

Edinburgh Consumer Group (1976) *Survey of Funeral Costs in Edinburgh.* Edinburgh: Edinburgh Consumer Group.

Eissler, K. (1955) *The Psychiatrist and the Dying Patient.* New York: International University Press.

Elfert, H. (1975) The nurse and the grieving patient. *Canadian Nurse 71 (2),* 30–1.

Ellard, J. *et al.* (1973) *Normal and Pathological Responses to Bereavement.* New York: MSS Information Corporation.

Emmet, D. (1966) *Rules, Roles and Relations.* London: Macmillan.

—— (1967) Ethics and the social worker in *Social Work and Social Values* (ed. Younghusband). Allen & Unwin.

Engelhardt, H. T. (1975) The counsels of finitude. *Hastings Center Report 5.*

English Citizens' Advice Bureaux Pamphlet (1975) *Practical Problems after a Death.*

Epstein, C. (1975) Nursing the dying patient, in *A–C–C.* Hemel Hempstead: Prentice Hall International. (See review in *Nursing Mirror* (31 July 1975) 74.)

Evans, B. (1976) The dying child. *World Med.* (March 24), 17–18.
Evans-Wentz, W. Y. (1960) *The Tibetan Book of the Dead.* Oxford University Press.
Fabian, J. How others die — reflections on the anthropology of death. *Social Research*, 543–67.
Farberow, N. L. (1963) *Taboo Topics.* New York: Otherton Press.
Feifel, H., ed. (1959) *The Meaning of Death.* New York: McGraw Hill.
Feifel, H., *et al.* (1967) Physicians consider death. *Proc. Am. Psychol. Assoc. Conv.*, 201–2.
Ference, T. P., *et al.* (1971) Priests and church: professionalisation of an organisation, in *The Professions and their Prospects* (ed. E. Friedson). London: Sage Publications.
Ferris, P. (1965, 1967) *The Doctors.* London: Penguin Books.
Flesch, R. (1975) A guide to interviewing the bereaved. *J. of Thanatol. 3 (2)*, 93–103.
Fletcher, G. (1968) Legal aspects of the decision not to prolong life. *J. of the Am. Med. Assoc. 203*, 65–8.
Fletcher, J. (1954) Euthanasia: our right to die, in *Morals and Medicine.* Boston: Beacon Press.
—— (1973) Ethics and euthanasia. *Am. J. of Nursing 73*, 671.
Fletcher, J. C. (1971) *Dialogue Between Medicine and Theology. Should Doctors Play God?* (Ed. C. A. Frazier.) Nashville: Broadman Press.
Fletcher, J. F. The right to live and the right to die. *Doc. in Med. Ethics 5* (SSME).
Flew, A. *Body, Mind and Death.* London: Macmillan.
Foot, P. (1977) Euthanasia. *Philosophy and Public Affairs 6*, 85–112.
Foren, R. & R. Bailey (1968) *Authority in Social Casework.* Pergamon Press.
Forester, A. C. (1976) Brain death and the donation of cadaver kidneys. *Health Bulletin*, 199–203.
Fox, R. The Samaritan contribution to suicide prevention. *Doc. in Med. Ethics 1* (SSME).
Freeman, J. M. & R. E. Cooke (1972) Is there a right to die — quickly? *J. of Pediatrics 80*, 904–8.
Freireich, E. J. (1972) The best medical care for the 'hopeless' patient. *Med. Opinion* Feb., 51–5.
French, J. & D. R. Schwartz (1973) Terminal care at home in two cultures. *Am. J. of Nursing 73*, 502–5.
Freidson, E. (1970 & 1975) *Profession of Medicine.* New York: Dodd, Mead.
Freud, S. (1917) Mourning and melancholia. *Standard Edition 14.*
Fuerst *et al.* (1974) *Fundamentals of Nursing.* Chapter 31. Philadelphia.
Fulton, R., ed. (1965) *Death and Identity.* New York: Wiley.
—— (1977) *Death, Grief and Bereavement: A Bibliography 1845–1975.* New York: Arno Press.
Gardener, R. F. R. (1975) A new ethical approach to abortion and its implications for the euthanasia dispute. *J. of Med. Ethics 1/3*, 127.
Gatch, M. McC. (1969) Death: Meaning and Mortality in *Christian Thoughts and Contemporary Culture.* New York: Seabury Press.
Geizhals, J. S. (1975) Attitudes toward death and dying: a study of occupational therapists and nurses. *J. of Thanatol. 3*, 243–69.
Gerber, I. (1975) Sequelae of anticipation of bereavement on the elderly survivor. *J. of Thanatol. 3 (1–2)*, 31–4.
Gibson, R. (1974) Caring for the bereaved. *Nursing Mirror 139 (15)*, 65–6.
Gifford, S. (1971) Freud's theories of unconscious immortality and the death instinct. *J. of Thanatol. 1*, 109–27.

Selected Bibliography

Glaser, B. & A. L. Strauss (1965) *Awareness of Dying*. Chicago: Aldine Press.
—— (1968) *Time for Dying*. Chicago: Aldine Press.
Glover, J. (1972) Not striving to keep alive. *Doc. in Med. Ethics 1* (SSME).
—— (1977) *Causing Death and Saving Lives*. London: Penguin Books.
Goldberg, I. K., *et al*, eds (1973) *Psychopharmacologic Agents for the Terminally Ill and Bereaved*. New York: Columbia University Press.
Goldfogel, L. (1970) Working with parents of a dying child. *Am. J. of Nursing 70*, 1677.
Goldstein, H. (1973) *Social Work Practice: A Unitary Approach*. S. Carolina.
Gorer, G. (1965) *Death, Grief and Mourning in Contemporary Britain*. London: Cresset.
Gorowitz, S., *et al*. (1976) *Moral Problems in Medicine*. Englewood Cliffs: Prentice Hall.
Gottheil, E., *et al*. (1976) Is it right to joke with a dying man? *Prism 2*.
Gould, J. & Lord Craigmyle, eds (1973) *Your Death Warrant? The Implications of Euthanasia*. New York: Arlington House.
Gruman, G. J. (1973) An historical introduction to ideas about voluntary euthanasia: with a bibliographic survey and guides for interdisciplinary studies. *Omega 4*, 87–138.
Gurney, E. J. (1972) Is there a right to die? A study of the law of euthanasia. *Cumberland Samford Law Review 3*, 235–61.
Gusterson, F. R. (1975) Personal view (to tell or not to tell). *BMJ* (6 December).
Gyulay, J. A. (1975) The forgotten grievers. *Am. J. of Nursing 75* (9), 1476–9.
Habgood, J. S. Euthanasia — a Christian view. *Doc. in Med. Ethics 5* (SSME).
Hagan, J. M. (1974) Infant deaths: nursing interaction and intervention with grieving families. *Nursing Forum 13* (4), 371–85.
Halley, M. M., *et al*. (1968) Definition of death. *New Eng. J. of Med. 279*, 834.
Halmos, P. (1965) *The Faith of the Counsellors*. London: Constable.
Hancock, S., *et al*. (1973) Care of the dying. *BMJ (January 6)*, 29–41.
Hanganu, E. & G. Popa (1977) Cancer and truth. *J. of Med. Ethics 3* (2).
Hankoff, L. D. (1975) Ancient Egyptian attitudes towards death and suicide. *The PHAROS April*, 60–4.
Harkess, R. *Omega: Who takes Care?* (Unpublished) Edinburgh Rotary Association.
Healy, E. F. (1956) *Medical Ethics*. Chicago: Loyola University Press.
Hendin, D. (1973) *Death as a Fact of Life*. New York: Norton.
Hertzberg, L. J. (1972) Cancer and the dying patient. *Am. J. of Psychiatry 128* (*Jan.*), 806–10.
High, D. M. (1972) Death: its conceptual elusiveness. *Soundings 55*, 438–58.
Hill, M. (1973) *A Sociology of Religion*. London: Heinemann.
Hinton, J. (1967/72) *Dying*. London: Penguin Books.
—— Patients' attitudes to dying. *Doc. in Med. Ethics 1* (SSME).
Hockey, L., ed (1976) *Women in Nursing*. London: Hodder & Stoughton.
Hollings, M. (1976) *Alive to Death*. Mayhew-McCrimmon.
Hollis, F. (1967) Principles and assumptions underlying casework practice, in *Social Work and Social Values* (ed. Younghusband).
Hostler, D. (1977) The right to live. *J. of Med. Ethics 3* (3).
Hunt, J. M., *et al*. (1977) Patients with protracted pain: a survey conducted at The London Hospital. *J. of Med. Ethics 3* (2).

Illich, I. (1974) The political uses of natural death. *Hastings Center Studies 2*, 3–20.
—— (1975) Clinical damage, medical monopoly, the expropriation of health: three dimensions of iatrogenic tort. *J. of Med. Ethics 1*, 78–80.
—— (1975) The medicalization of life. *J. of Med. Ethics 1/2*, 73–7.
—— (1975) *Medical Nemesis: The Expropriation of Health.* London: Trinity Press.
Incurable Patients Bill (1976) *Hansard 368. 196.* London: HMSO.
Ingelfinger, F. J. (1973) Bedside ethics for the hopeless case. *New Eng. J. of Med. 289*, 914–15.
Irvine, E. (1964) The right to intervene. *Social Work (U.K.) 21 (2).*
Isaacs, B., *et al.* (1971) The concept of pre-death. *Lancet 1*, 1115.
Jackson, P. L. (1974) Chronic grief. *Am. J. of Nursing 74 (7)*, 1288–91.
—— (1975) The child's developing concept of death. *Nursing Forum 14 (2)*, 204–15.
Jarvis, P. (1976: 2) A sociological analysis of the doctrines of the ministry and ordination. *Contact 53.*
—— (1976: 3) The potential resignee from the ministry. *Contact 54.*
J.B.C.N.S. (1976) Care of the dying. *Nursing Mirror: Nursing Care Supplement 143 (8).*
Jellinek, M. (1976) Erosion of patient trust in large medical centers. *Hastings Center Report 6*, 16–19.
Jennett, B. (1975) The donor doctor's dilemma: observations on the recognition and management of brain death. *J. of Med. Ethics 1*, 63–6.
—— (1977) Diagnosis of brain death. *J. of Med. Ethics 3*, 4–5.
Kahana, B. & E. Kahana (1972) Attitudes of young men and women toward awareness of death. *Omega 3*, 37–44.
Kao, C. C. L. (1976) Maturity and paternalism in health care. *Ethics in Sci. and Med. 3*, 179–86.
Kastenbaum, R. & R. Aisenberg (1975) *The Psychology of Death.* London: Duckworth.
Katz, J. & A. M. Capron (1975) *Catastrophic Diseases: Who Decides What?* New York: Russell Sage Foundation.
Kaufman, C. (1959) Existentialism and death. *Chicago Review XIII*, 75–93.
Kelly, G. (1950) The duty of using artificial means of preserving life. *Theological Studies 11*, 203–20.
Kennedy, I. (1973) The legal definition of death. *Medico-Legal J. 41*, 36.
—— (1976) The legal effect of requests by the terminally ill and aged not to receive further treatment from doctors. *Criminal Law Review.*
—— (1976) The Karen Quinlan case: problems and proposals. *J. of Med. Ethics 2*, 3–7.
—— (1977) When the dying ask to die, can death be denied them? *The Listener*, 14th July.
—— (1977) The definition of death. *J. of Med. Ethics 3 (1).*
Keywood, O. (1974) Care of the dying in their own home, *Nursing Times 70 (39)*, 1516–17.
Klein, D. F. Methodology for study of bereavement. *J. of Thanatol. 2 (3–4)*, 765–867.
Kluge, E.-H. (1975) *The Practice of Death.* New Haven: Yale University Press.
Kobrzycki, P. (1975) Dying with dignity at home. *Am. J. of Nursing 75 (8)*, 1312–13.
Koenig, R. (1973) Dying versus well-being. *Omega 4*, 181–94.

Selected Bibliography

Krupp, G. R. & B. Kilgfeld (1966) The bereaved reaction, a cross-cultural evaluation. *J. of Relig. and Health 1* (*3*), 222–46.

Kübler-Ross, E. (1970) *On Death and Dying.* Tavistock Publications.

—— (1975) *Death as the Final Stage of Growth.* New Jersey: Prentice-Hall.

Kutscher, A. H., ed. (1969) *But not to Lose: A Book for Comfort for those Bereaved.* New York: Frederick Fell Inc.

—— (1969) *Death and Bereavement.* Springfield, Illinois: Charles C. Thomas.

—— (1969) *A Bibliography of Books on Death, Bereavement, Loss and Grief 1955–1968.* New York: Health Sciences Publishing Corporation.

Kutscher, A. H., *et al. Communicating Issues in Thanatology.* New York: MSS Information Corp.

Kutscher, A. H. & M. R. Goldberg (1973) *Caring for the Dying Patient and His Family: a Model for Medical Education–Medical Center Conferences.* New York: Health Sciences Publishing Corp.

Lacasse, C. M. (1975) A dying adolescent. *Am. J. of Nursing 74,* 1067.

Lamerton, R. C. (1974) The need for hospices. *Nursing Times 71* (*4*), 155–7.

—— (1977) Going deeper into care of the dying. *Nursing Mirror 144* (*9*), 64–5.

Lasagna, L. (1975) *The Conflict of Interest Between Physician as Therapist and Experimenter.* Philadelphia: Society for Health and Human Values.

Laws, E. H., *et al.* Views on euthanasia. *Doc. in Med. Ethics 5* (SSME).

Leared, J. (1974) The Camden bereavement project. *Midwife and Health Visitor 10* (*1*), 15–16.

Lester, D. (1971) Attitudes toward death today and thirty-five years ago. *Omega 2,* 168.

Lester, D., *et al.* (1974) Attitudes of nursing students and nursing faculty toward death. *Nursing Research 23* (*1*), 50–3.

Levy, B., *et al.* (1976) The doctor and the dying role. *The Practitioner 216.*

Levy, B. & A. Balfour Sclare (1976) A study of bereavement in general practice. *J. of R. Coll. of General Practitioners 26,* 329–36.

Lewis, C. S. (1961) *A Grief Observed.* London: Faber and Faber.

Lewis, R. & A. Maude (1952) *Professional People.* London: Phoenix House Ltd.

Lifton, R. J. & E. Olson (1975) *Living and Dying.* Wildwood House.

Lock, S. & R. C. Lamerton (1975) *The Hour of Death.* London: Geoffrey Chapman.

Keith-Lucas, A. (1963) A critique of the principle of client self-determination. *Social Work (U.S.A.) 8* (*3*).

McFarlane, J. K. (1976) A charter for caring. *J. of Advanced Nursing 1,* 187–196.

McGilloway, F. A. (1976) Dependence and vulnerability in the nurse/patient situation. *J. of Advanced Nursing 1,* 229–36.

Macguire, D. (1972) The freedom to die. *Commonweal 96,* 423–7.

Mackenzie, N. (1971) *The Professional Ethic and the Hospital Service.* The English Universities Press Ltd.

McKeown, T. (1965) *Medicine and Culture.* London: Wellcome Institute of the History of Medicine.

MacLean, U. (1974) *Nursing in Contemporary Society.* London: Routledge.

Maddison, D. & B. Raphael. Normal bereavement as an illness requiring care: psychopharmacological approaches. *J. of Thanatol. 2* (*3–4*), 785–820.

Magee, B. (1977) *Facing Death.* London: William Kimber.

Magraw, R. M. (1973) Grief: its clinical importance and its resolution. *Modern Medicine,* October.

Maguire, D. C. (1974) *The Future of Death.* New York: Doubleday & Co., Inc.

Malone, R. J. (1974) Is there a right to a natural death? *New Eng. Law Review 9*, 293–310.

Man and Medicine (1975) *The Journal of Values and Ethics in Health Care 1.* New York: Columbia University College of Physicians & Surgeons.

Manson, H. H. (1972) Justifying the final solution. *Omega 3*, 79–87.

Marinker, M. (1975) Why make people patients? *J. of Med. Ethics 1*, 81–4.

Marks, M. J. (1976) Dealing with death: the grieving patient and family. *Am. J. of Nursing 76* (9), 1488–91.

Martin, D. (1967) *A Sociology of English Religion.* London: Heinemann.

Masters, R. D. (1975) Is contract an adequate basis for medical ethics? *Hastings Center Report 5.*

May, W. F. (1971) On not facing death alone. *Hastings Center Report 1*, 8–9.

—— (1973) Attitudes toward the newly dead. *Hastings Center Studies 1 (1)*, 3–13.

—— (1975) Code, covenant, contract or philanthropy. *Hastings Center Report 5.*

Mervyn, F. (1971) The plight of dying patients in hospitals. *Am. J. of Nursing 71*, 1988–90.

Meyer, B. C. (1969) Truth and the physician. *Bull. of the New York Acad. of Med. 45*, 59–71.

Miller, H. (1973) *Medicine and Society.* Oxford University Press.

Mitchell, B. (1976) Is a moral consensus in medical ethics possible? *J. of Med. Ethics 2*, 18–23.

Mitchell, P. H. (1973) *Concepts Basic to Nursing*, pp. 145–8. New York: McGraw-Hill.

Mitton, C. L., ed. (1972) *The Social Sciences and the Churches.* Edinburgh: T. & T. Clark.

Montange, C. H. (1974) Informed consent and the dying patient. *Yale Law Journal 83*, 1632–64.

Montefiore, H. W., *et al.* (1973) *Death Anxiety — Normal and Pathological Aspects.* New York: MSS Information Corporation.

Moore, F. D. (1968) Medical responsibility for the prolongation of life. *J. of the Am. Med. Assoc. 206*, 384–6.

Morison, R. S. & L. Kass (1971) Death — process or event? *Science 173*, 694–702.

Morison, R. S. (1973) Dying. *Sci. Am. 229*, 55–62.

Moser, M. J. (1975) Death in Chinese: a two-dimensional analysis. *J. of Thanatol. 3*, 169–85.

Murray, J. T., *et al.* (1974) A study of the contribution of the health visitor to the support and care of terminally ill patients and their relatives. *Health Bulletin 32* (6), 250–2.

Murray, M. (1976) *Fundamentals of Nursing*, chapter 28. New Jersey: Prentice-Hall.

Neale, R. E. (1973) *The Art of Dying.* New York: Harper & Row.

Needham, A. (1971) Talking it over. *Nursing Mirror*, 15 January.

Nelson, J. (1976) Live thoughts on dying patients. *Nursing Times*, 15 April, 592–3.

Nichaolson, R. (1975) Should the patient be allowed to die. *J. of Med. Ethics 1/1*, 5–9.

Nighswonger, C. A. (1971) Ministry to the dying as a learning encounter. *J. of Thanatol. 1*, 101–8.

Northrup, F. C. (1974) The dying child. *American Journal of Nursing 74*, 1067.

211

Selected Bibliography

Noyes, R. & T. A. Travis (1973) The care of terminally ill patients. *Archives of Internal Med. 132*, 607–11.
Nuffield Provincial Hospitals Trust (1972) *A Symposium of Introspections* (ed. G. McLachlan). London: Oxford University Press.
Nursing Mirror (1974) Symposium on care of the dying. 10 October, 53–70.
Nursing Times (1976) Care of the dying. (Reprint Publication: MacMillan Journals Ltd.)
Palmer, I. O. (1976) Discussing death. *Nursing Times 72* (7), 261.
Papal Allocution to a Congress of Anaesthetists (1957) *Acta Apostolicas Sedis* (*24 Nov.*), 1027–33.
Pappworth, M. H. (1967) *Human Guinea Pigs*. London: Routledge.
Parkes, C. M. (1964) Effects of bereavement on physical and mental health — a study of the medical records of widows. *B.M.J. 2*, 274–9.
—— (1964) Grief as an illness. *New Society 3* (*80*), 11.
—— (1972) Accuracy of predictions of survival in later stages of cancer. *B.M.J. 2*, 29–31.
—— (1972) *Bereavement*. London: Penguin Books.
—— The patient's right to know the truth. *Proc. of the R. Soc. of Med. 66*, 536.
Parsons, T. (1951) *The Social System*. Illinois: The Free Press.
—— (1954) *Essays in Sociological Theory*. Illinois: Free Press.
Patey, E. H. (1975) Matters of life and death: to care — or to kill. *Nursing Mirror, 2 October*, 40–41.
Pearson, L. ed. (1969) *Death and Dying: Current Issues in the Treatment of the Dying Person*. New York: Jason Aronson Inc.
Pells, J. (1974) Prolonging life. *Nursing Times 70* (*8*), 21 Feb., 21 *and* 28 March.
Peretz, D. *et al.* (1971) A survey of physicians' attitudes toward death and bereavement. *J. of Thanatol. 1*, 91–100.
Pine, V. R. (1975) Institutionalised communication about dying and death. *J. of Thanatol. 3* (*1–2*), 1–12.
Pincus, L. (1975) How to help the bereaved. *Social Work Today 6* (*13*), 392.
—— (1976) *Death and the Family*. London: Faber and Faber.
Pius XII (1957) The Pope speaks, prolongation of life. *Osservatore Romano 4*, 393–8.
Platt, M. (1975) Looking at the body. *Hastings Center Report 5*.
—— (1975) On asking to die. *Hastings Center Report 5/6*, 9–10.
Potter, R. B. (1968) The paradoxical preservation of principle. *Villanova Law Review 13*, 784–92.
Powledge, T. M., *et al.* (1975) The 'duty' to preserve life. *Hastings Center Report 5/2*, 14–21.
Poynter, F. N. L., ed. (1969) *Medicine and Culture*. London: Wellcome Institute of the History of Medicine.
Poynter, N. (1971) *Medicine and Man*. London: Penguin Books.
Prichard, E. R. (1972) Planning for the terminally ill patient: the S.W.'s responsibility. *J. of Thanatol. 2* (*1–2*).
Proceedings of a National Symposium. (1972) D.H.S.S. — care of the dying. *Report on Health and Social Subjects 5*. London: HMSO.
Quarnstrom, U. (1978) *Patients' Reactions to Impending Death*. Taby, Sweden: Ulla Quarnstrom.
Quint, J. C. (1967) *The Nurse and the Dying Patient*. New York: Macmillan.
Rachels, J. (1975) Active and passive euthanasia. *New Eng. J. of Med. 292*, 78–80.
—— (1975) Study suggests new less rigid criteria for declaring death. *Med. World News 16*, 26–7.

Raglan, Lord (1972) The case for voluntary euthanasia. *Doc. in Med. Ethics 1* (SSME).

Ramsay, P. (1970) *The Patient as a Person*. New Haven: Yale University Press.

Ramsey, I. T. Moral problems facing the medical profession at the present time. *Doc. in Med. Ethics 1* (SSME).

Raphael, D. D. (1967) *Political Theory and the Rights of Man*. London: Macmillan.

Raven, R. W., ed. (1975) *The Dying Patient*. London: Pitman Medical.

Rees, W. D. & S. G. Lutkins (1967) Mortality of bereavement. *B.M.J. 4*, 13–16.

Report of the Working Party on *Elderly People at Risk*. (1974) Age Concern, Scotland. November.

Reynolds, D. K. & N. L. Farberow (1976) *Suicide Inside and Out*. Berkeley: University of California Press.

Richardson, Sir J., Lord P. C. Edmund-Davies & D. Coggan, Archbishop of Canterbury (1977) Edwin Stevens Lecture. On dying and dying well. *R. Soc. of Med. 70*.

Robitscher, J. (1972) The right to die. *Hastings Center Report 11–14*.

Rogers, J. & M. L. S. Vachon (1975) Nurses can help the bereaved. *Canadian Nurse 71 (6)*, 16–19.

Roper, N. (1973) *Principles of Nursing*, chapter 4. Edinburgh: Churchill Livingstone.

Ross, E. K. (1971) What is it like to be dying? *Am. J. of Nursing 71*, 54–61.

Royal College of Nursing (1976). Code of Professional Conduct

Rudikoff, S. The problem of euthanasia. *Doc. in Med. Ethics 5* (SSME).

Russell, O. R. (1975) *Freedom to Die: Moral and Legal Aspects of Euthanasia*. New York: Human Sciences Press.

Sackett, W. W. (1969) Death with dignity. *Med. Opinion and Review 5*, 25–31.

Sartre, J.P. (1969) *Being and Nothingness*. London: Methuen.

Saunders, C. M. S. (1959) Care of the dying. *Nursing Times 55*, 9, 16, 23, 30 Oct., 6, 13 Nov.

—— (1963) The treatment of intractable pain in terminal cancer. *Proc. of the R. Soc. of Med. 56*, 191–7.

—— (1967) The care of the terminal stages of cancer. *Ann. of the R. Coll. of Surg. of Eng. 41* Supplement, 162–9.

—— (1969) The moment of truth: care of the dying person, in *Death and Dying* (ed. L. Pearson), pp. 49–78. Cleveland: Case Western Reserve University Press.

—— The care of the dying patient and his family. *Doc. in Med. Ethics 1* (SSME).

—— (1976) Care of the dying. *Nursing Times 1*, 8, 15, 22, 29 July and 5, 12 August.

Schmale, A. H., Jnr. Normal grief is not a disease. *J. of Thanatol. 2 (3–4)*, 785–820.

Schnafer, N., *et al.* (1973) *Management of the Dying Patient and his Family*. New York: MSS Information Corporation.

Schoenberg, B. C. & Peretz, eds (1970) *Loss and Grief: Psychological Management in Medical Practice*. New York: Columbia University Press.

Schoolman, H. M. (1977) The role of the physician as patient advocate. *New Eng. J. of Med. 296*, 103–5.

Selected Bibliography

Schowalter, J. E. (1971) Death and the pediatric nurse. *J. of Thanatol. 1*, 81–9.

—— (1975) Pediatric nurses dream of death. *J. of Thanatol. 3*, 223–31.

Schultz, R. & D. Aderman (1974) Clinical research and the stages of dying. *Omega 5*, 134–43.

—— (1976) How the medical staff copes with dying patients: a critical review. *Omega 1*, 11–21.

Scott, B. T. (1974) Doctors and dying. Is euthanasia becoming accepted? *Med. Opinion*, May, 31–4.

Scott, C. E. (1972) Reflections on dying. *Soundings 55*, 472–9.

Scottish Citizens' Advice Bureaux Pamphlet. (1975) *Practical Problems After a Death*. Scottish Citizens' Advice Bureaux.

Seitz, P. M. & L. H. Warrick (1974) Perinatal death: the grieving mother. *Am. J. of Nursing 74 (11)*, 2028–33.

Sheskin, A. & S. E. Wallace (1976) Differing bereavements: suicide, natural and accidental death. *Omega 7 (3)*, 229–42.

Shotter, E. F. (1970) *Matters of Life and Death*. London.

Shusterman, L. R. (1973) Death and dying: a critical review of the literature. *Nursing Outlook 21*, 465–71.

Siegler, M. & H. Osmond (1976) The doctor and the dying role. *The Practitioner 216*, 690–4.

Silving, H. (1954) Euthanasia: a study in comparative criminal law. *Univ. of Pennsylvania Law Review 103*, 350–89.

Simpson, M. A. (1976) Brought in dead. *Omega 7 (3)*, 243–8.

Skillmann, J. J. (1974) Ethical dilemmas in the care of the critically ill. *The Lancet 11*, 634–7.

Slater, E. Assisted suicide. Some ethical considerations. *Doc. in Med. Ethics 5* (SSME).

Slater, E. *et al.* (1976) *Death with Dignity*. London: The Voluntary Euthanasia Society.

Smith, D. H. (1976) *The Sanctity of Social Life: Physicians and the Critically Ill*.

Snyder, M. *et al.* (1973) Changes in nursing students' attitudes towards death and dying. *Int. J. of Soc. Psychiatry 19 (3/4)*, 214–18.

Sobran, M. J., Jr. (1976) The right to die (I). *The Human Life Review 2*, 27–32.

Solnit, A. & S. Provences, eds (1963) *Modern Perspective in Child Development Part II The Child's Reaction to the Fear of Dying*. New York: International Universities Press.

Sonstegard, L. (1976) Dealing with death; the grieving nurse. *Am. J. of Nursing 76 (9)*, 1490–2.

Spanton, J. (1976) Coping with death. *Nursing Times 72 (19)*, 741.

Spencer, T. E. (1975) Cremation and life style. *J. of Thanatol. 3*, 35–42.

Starr, S. (1975) 'I'm going to die . . .'. *Nursing Times 71 (18)*.

Starrs, A. (1976) *Geriatric Nursing*. London: Baillière Tindall.

Steinfels, P. & R. M. Veatch (1975) *Death Inside Out*. New York: Harper & Row.

Stengel, E. (1970) *Suicide and Attempted Suicide*. Harmondsworth: Pelican Books.

Stephen, S. (1972) *Death Comes Home*. London, Oxford: Mowbray.

Stevens, R. (1966) *Medical Practice in Modern England*. New Haven: Yale University Press.

Stevenson, C. L. (1944/62) *Ethics and Language*. New Haven: Yale University Press.

Stewart, A. M. (1975) Cot deaths. *Nursing Mirror 11 December*, 57–8.
Stewart, D. W. (1975) Religious correlates of the fear of death. *J. of Thanatol. 3*, 161–4.
Strank, R. A. (1972) Caring for the chronic sick and dying: a study of attitudes. *Nursing Times 10 February*, 166–9.
Strauss, A. L., *et al.* (1964) The nonaccountability of terminal care. *Hospitals 38*, 73–87.
Sudnow, D. (1960) *Passing On: The Social Organization of Dying*. New Jersey: Prentice-Hall.
Symposium (Wilkes, etc.) (1974) Care of the dying. *Nursing Mirror, 10 Oct.*
Szasz, T. S. (1971) The ethics of suicide. *The Antioch Review 31*, 7–17.
Templer, D. I. (1970) The construction of validation of a death anxiety scale. *J. of General Psychology 82*, 163–77.
—— Death anxiety scale (1969) *Proc. 77th Annual Conv. of the Am. Psychology Assoc. 4*, 737–8.
Templer, D. I. & C. F. Ruff (1975) The relation between death anxiety and religion in psychiatric patients. *J. of Thanatol.*
Thompson, G. The euthanasia debate. *Doc. in Med. Ethics 2* (SSME).
Thompson, I. E. (1976) Suicide and philosophy. *Contact 54.*
—— (1976) Implications of medical ethics. *J. of Med. Ethics 2*, 74–82.
Thompson, M. R. Communication with patient and relatives. (Unpublished paper.) Chaplain Royal Marsden Hospital.
Thorley, A. The quality of death. *Doc. in Med. Ethics 2* (SSME).
Tillich, P. (1952) *The Courage to Be*. New Haven: Yale University Press.
Timms, N. (1970) *Social Work — An Outline for the Intending Student*. London.
Titmuss, R. (1970) *The Gift Relationship*. London: Penguin Books.
Torrie, M. (1970) *Begin Again*. London: J. M. Dent & Son.
Towler, R. (1969) The social status of the Anglican minister, in *Sociology of Religion* (ed. R. Robertson). London: Penguin.
Toynbee, A. (1968–9) *Man's Concern with Death*. London: Hodder & Stoughton.
Troisfontaines, R. (1965) *I do not die*. New York: Desclee.
Trowell, H., ed. (1971) *The Unfinished Debate on Euthanasia*. London: Institute of Religion and Medicine.
Twycross, R. G. A plea for Eu Thanatos. *Doc. in Med. Ethics 2* (SSME).
—— (1975) Relief of terminal pain. *B.M.J. 4*, 212.
—— (1975) The use of narcotic analgesics in terminal *illness. J. of Med. Ethics 1/1*, 10–17.
Veatch, R. M. (1972) Brain death: welcome definition or dangerous judgment? *Hastings Center Report 2*, 10–13.
—— (1975) Medical ethics in a revolutionary age. *J. of Current Soc. Issues 12*, 4–19.
—— (1975) The whole brain-oriented concept of death: an outmoded philosophical formulation. *J. of Thanatol. 3 (1–12)*, 13–30.
—— (1976) *Death, Dying and Biological Revolution*. New Haven: Yale University Press.
Versius, N. (1970) Social misconception of death. *Concilium 5 (7).*
Vickery, K. O. A. Medicated survival—the press, the public, the professions and the patient. *Doc. in Med. Ethics 5* (SSME).
Voluntary Euthanasia Society (1970) *A Plea for Legislation to Permit Voluntary Euthanasia*. London.
Voluntary Euthanasia Society (1976) *Death with Dignity*. London.
Ward, A. W. M. (1976) Mortality of bereavement. *B.M.J., March 20.*

Selected Bibliography

Wardron, F. E. (1957) The acceptance of dependency in social casework. *Case Conference 4 (6).*

Wassmer, T. A. (1968) Between life and death: ethical and moral issues involved in recent medical advances. *Villanova Law Review 13,* 759–83.

Weightman, G. (1977) Death and the doctors. *New Society 4 August.*

Weiner, A. The use of psychopharmacological agents in the management of the bereaved. *J. of Thanatol. 2 (3–4),* 785–820.

Weisman, A. D. (1972) *On Dying and Denying, a Psychiatric Study of Terminality.* New York: Behavioural Publications Inc.

Weller, M. F. (1975) Bereavement. *Health Visitor 48 (5),* 155–6.

White, D. (1972) Death control. *New Society 22,* 502–5.

White, P., ed. (1969) Care of patients with fatal illness. *Ann. of the New York Acad. of Sci. 164,* 635–896.

Wielgus, K. (1976) Custodial and therapeutic patient relationships. *Ethics in Sci. and Med. 3,* 71–94.

Wilkes, E. (1965) Terminal cancer at home. *Lancet i,* 799–801.

Williams, G. (1957) *The Sanctity of Life and the Criminal Law.* New York: Alfred Knopf Inc.

—— (1973) Euthanasia. *Medico-Legal Journal.*

Williams, J. Death and bereavement. Age Concern, Eng. *Manifesto Series 17.*

Williams, R. H. (1969) Our role in the generation modification and termination of life. *J. of the Am. Med. Assoc. 209,* 914–17.

Wilson, F. G. (1971) Social isolation and bereavement. *Nursing Times, 4 March,* 269.

Wilson, M. (1975) Communication with the dying. *J. of Med. Ethics 1/1,* 18–21.

—— (1975) *Health is for People.* London: Darton, Longman and Todd.

Winget, C., et al. (1977) Attitudes towards euthanasia. *J. of Med. Ethics 3 (8),* 25.

Winter, A., ed. (1965) *The Moment of Death: A Symposium.* Springfield, Illinois: Charles C. Thomas.

Wise, D. J. (1974) Learning about dying. *Nursing Outlook 22 (1),* 42–4.

Worcester, A. (1961) *The Care of the Aging, the Dying and the Dead.* Springfield, Illinois: Charles C. Thomas.

Yeaworth, R. C., et al. (1974) Attitudes of nursing students towards the dying patient. *Nursing Research 23 (1),* 20–24.

Yondorf, B. (1975) The declining and wretched. *Public Policy XXII,* 465–82.

Young, M., et al. (1963) The mortality of widowers. *Lancet ii,* 454–6.

Zahourek, R. & J. S. Jensen (1973) Grieving and the loss of the newborn. *Am. J. of Nursing 73,* 836–9.

Zinner, E. S. (1971) A proposal: developing the role of the clinical associate in the field of terminal patient care. *J. of Thanatol. 1 (3),* 156–71.

Zola, I. K. (1972) Medicine as an institution of social control. *The Soc. Review 20,* 487–504.

Zorab, J. S. M. (1975) The definition of death and its clinical significance. *World Medicine, December 3.*

Index

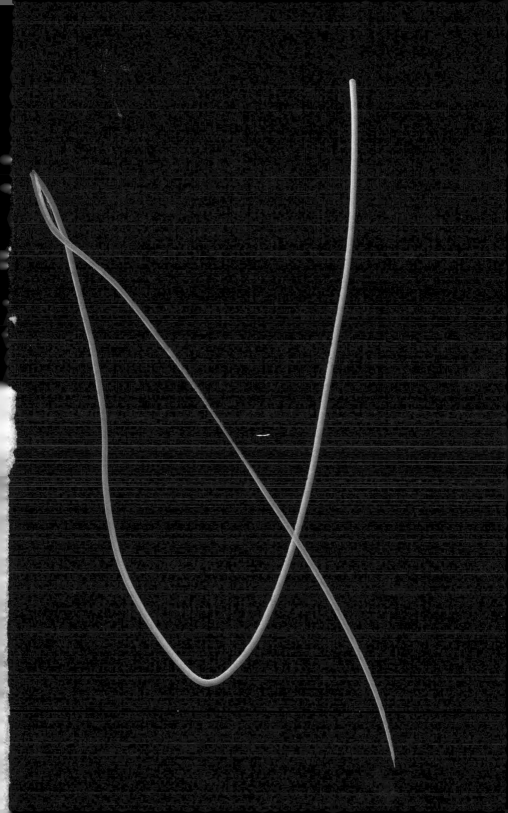

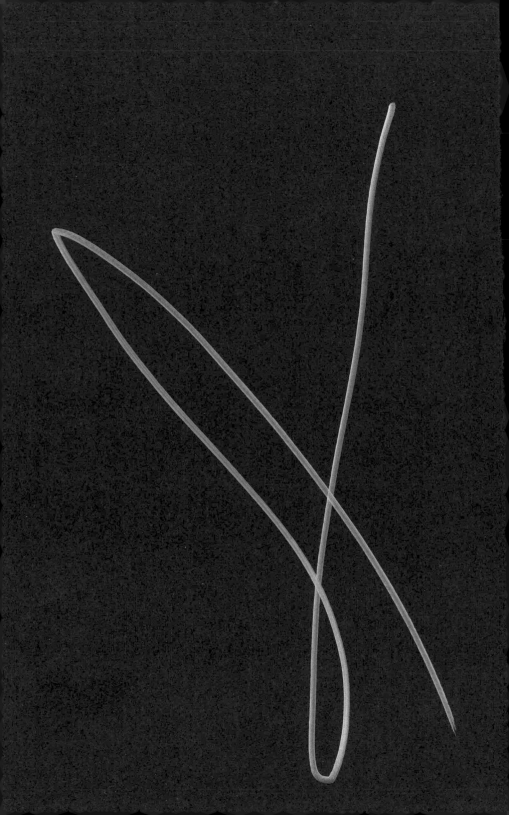